The Complete
Home
Medical Guide
for Cats

STEPHEN SCHNECK AND DR. NIGEL NORRIS

The Complete Home Medical Guide for Cats

STEIN AND DAY/*Publishers*/ New York

First published, 1976
Copyright © 1976 by Stephen Schneck
All rights reserved
Designed by David Miller
Printed in the United States of America
Stein and Day/*Publishers*/Scarborough House,
Briarcliff Manor, N.Y. 10510

SECOND PRINTING 1976

Library of Congress Cataloging in Publication Data

Schneck, Stephen, 1933–
    The complete home medical guide for cats.

    I. Cats—Diseases. I. Norris, Nigel, joint author.
II. Title.
SF985.S36   636.8'08'96024   74-31109
ISBN 0-8128-1797-4

Introduction

One of the many problems facing veterinaries is how to explain, in non-technical language, what is wrong with a pet animal so that the owner can understand and, if possible, help the healing process. The layman can only be expected to have a superficial knowledge of anatomy and physiology, and the rapid advances in diagnosis and treatment in recent years have made the gulf between professional advisor and client even wider.

Veterinarians in small-animal practice soon gain experience in explaining, as simply as possible, what may be a very complex condition. Nevertheless, most of us have felt the need for an up-to-date book compiled especially for the pet owner.

The Complete Home Medical Guide for Cats, written by a pet owner in collaboration with a practicing veterinarian, neatly fills this gap. Factually correct, the information is presented in clear everyday language which will give useful guidance to even the most inexperienced owner with little or no knowledge of biology.

In many parts of the world, a dog or cat owner may be far from the nearest veterinary, and though in some countries flying doctor services are available, the "flying vet" is, as yet, a luxury pet owners cannot afford. In these remote areas antibiotics and other medicines are available, but they are of little use without some knowledge and advice on how to use them. In the United Kingdom and the United States, as well as in many other countries, antibiotics, etc. are (quite rightly) sold only on prescription. There are, however, many simple and effective remedies which can be used before professional advice is sought, or when it is not possible to get immediate treatment from a vet. This book helps the owner to cope with both situations and also gives the basic rules for prompt and effective first-aid in emergencies.

Veterinarians, of course, are most concerned that people should look after their pets in a responsible way. This means caring for the health and welfare of the animal and being alert for any changes which may be signs of impending illness. *The Complete Home Medical Guide for Cats* should be of considerable help in furthering this aim and will, I am sure, be welcomed by both pet owners and veterinarians.

Henry Carter, MRCVS

Past President

British Small Animal Veterinary Association

How to Use
This Book

Successful home medical treatment is based on the ability to make the correct medical diagnosis. A sick or injured animal exhibits certain symptoms. These symptoms are signs which, properly observed, lead to an intelligent and informed diagnosis.

This book has been specially designed to help the responsible pet owner make this diagnosis.

Every symptom likely to be exhibited by a sick or injured animal is listed in the Index. There is also a Table of Contents which lists the entries according to the parts of the body affected. If, for example, the animal is suffering from ear mites (Otodectic Mange) treatment for this condition will be found by referring to the Table of Contents under problems of Head and Neck. However, if the pet owner does not know that excessive scratching of the ear, shaking of the head, a discharge from the ear, or waxy, brown crusts in the ear suggests ear mites, any of these symptoms can be found in the Index and the reader will be

3

referred to the appropriate entry. If, as in this instance, home treatment is possible, this treatment will be described in the entry. When home treatment is not recommended, the entry will inform the reader.

Of course it is not always possible to make accurate diagnoses solely on the basis of simple observation. Many diseases can be diagnosed only by a veterinary with laboratory facilities.

No book, however informative, can substitute for professional treatment. What this book can do, is to inform the pet owner when a vet's services are necessary, what constitutes an emergency, and, in many cases, serve as a temporary paramedical aid when a vet is not immediately available.

Contents

2. PROBLEMS OF THE HEAD AND NECK

3. PROBLEMS OF THE SKIN AND HAIR

4. PROBLEMS OF THE CHEST

5. PROBLEMS OF THE ABDOMEN

9. PROBLEMS OF THE BACK

10. PROBLEMS AFFECTING THE WHOLE BODY

11. PROBLEMS OF FEMALE CATS ONLY

12. POISONING

The Complete
Home
Medical Guide
for Cats

1

General
Cat Care

Analgesics

Analgesics are pain relievers. When administering these pain killers pay careful attention to dosages; use them only when the cat is in obvious pain or acute discomfort. You should know your pet's normal behavior pattern to gauge the degree of pain accurately.

Dosage: One-half of a 250-mg. Tylenol ® tablet (or equivalent) per 10 pounds body weight, once a day. (See How to Administer Tablets and Pills.)

Warning: Never give your cat aspirin preparations; they have an adverse effect on the animal's bone marrow. Do not administer codeine preparations.

Anthropomorphism

Next to sheer ignorance, anthropomorphism is probably the second-ranking cause of improper home medical treatment. Anthropomorphism, in this context, is the fallacy of attributing human behavior and mentality to cats.

While it is perfectly normal to speak of an animal as being "nearly human," actually believing it can lead to serious errors in judgment which, in turn, can lead to incorrect medical treatment. If we think of a cat as a human being, we cannot properly observe and evaluate the animal's behavior. In many instances this attitude makes it impossible to reach a correct diagnosis.

Cats have their own psychology, their own behavior patterns, and their own set of reactions. To treat cats intelligently, we must think of them as cats, and not as four-legged people.

Antibiotics and Antibiotic Treatment

The use of antibiotics is beyond the proper scope of home treatment. Its inclusion here is meant to be informative rather than practical.

Antibiotics are drugs that kill or inhibit the growth of germs that cause infections. They are most effective when administered during the early growth stages of infections. (Antibiotics are usually ineffective against virus infections.)

Ideally, if your cat has an infectious disease, the particular strain of bacteria that is causing it should be identified and the specific antibiotic administered. Unfortunately, disease states are rarely ideal, so a broad-spectrum antibiotic may be administered while a specific germ is being identified.

If there is no response within twenty-four hours, another broad-spectrum antibiotic may be used, and possibly yet another, until a satisfactory response is obtained.

Artificial Respiration

Artificial respiration does the work of normal breathing, moving air into and out of the cat's lungs. Artificial respiration should be administered as soon as one observes that the animal is not breathing. A cat that has stopped breathing and whose cardiac activity has ceased for over five minutes will be beyond recovery.

Technique: Lay the cat on its right side. Open its mouth to make sure that there are no obstructions to breathing. If there are obstructions (e.g., sand, gravel), pull them out

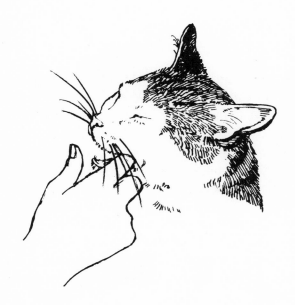

with your finger. Also be sure that the cat's tongue is clear of the back of the throat. It is possible to be bitten if a gag is not used. Place the flat of both hands below the shoulder

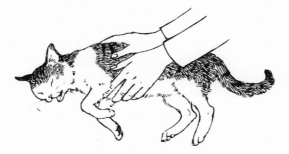

blade and over the ribs. Press down firmly to empty the lungs, release, and wait. The movements should be brisk

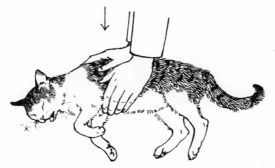

and forceful. Press down hard; release suddenly. The lungs

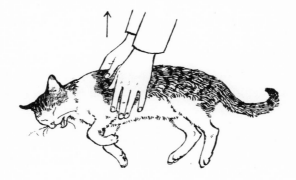

should fill as the chest wall returns to its normal position. Repeat pressing down and releasing the pressure every five seconds, until the cat is breathing on its own again.

Swinging technique: Slap the cat sharply on the side once or twice. Then lift the animal up by its hind legs, extend your arms, and swing it back and forth ten times.

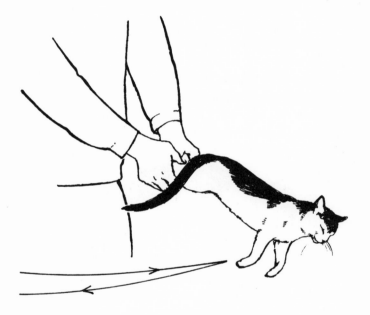

Wait a few seconds for a gasp. If there is none, swing the cat again.

When you swing a cat as described, the weight of the abdominal contents will contract and expand the lungs. If after four such swinging sessions the cat is still not breathing, administer mouth-to-nostril resuscitation. (You'll catch far fewer germs from kissing a cat than you'll get from kissing a person.)

Mouth-to-nostril resuscitation: Hold the cat's mouth closed and blow into its nostrils. Wait and allow the chest to empty; repeat. This simple procedure inflates the animal's lungs with air so that they can function normally again. If the cat does not respond immediately, remember, as long as you can hear a heartbeat, there is hope!

Automobile Accidents: Moving an Injured Cat

First consideration: Do not move the animal any more than you have to. Decide where you are going to move the cat before you move it.

Moving a cat in great pain is not the easiest thing to do, so be prepared for some problems. A badly hurt or badly frightened animal may bite or scratch anyone who tries to touch it, including its owner. Don't waste time trying to calm the cat with soothing talk; if it is really hurt, it will not hear you. Take the proper precautions against being bitten and get on with the job.

Precautions: The best way to prevent the animal from biting and scratching you while you are trying to move it is to cover it with a blanket or coat and then gently lift and carry the whole bundle of cat and coat. (See Transportation of Injured Cats.)

It is better and much faster to get the cat to the vet than to try to get the vet to the cat. If possible, have someone telephone the vet so that emergency treatment is ready when you arrive. If you do not know a vet, call the police; they can probably tell you where the cat should be taken.

Warmth, no fluids: Try to keep the cat warm while you are getting it to the vet. Do not apply external heat. To prevent loss of body heat, wrap the animal in a coat or a blanket. Do not try to numb the pain by pouring whisky down the cat's throat. Do not try to counteract shock with warm milk or water. This is to prevent vomiting if an anesthetic has to be administered.

Bleeding: If the cat is bleeding, try to stop or at least stanch the bleeding. Try to determine whether the bleeding is from an artery or a vein (arterial or venous). This is done by observing the way the blood flows.

If the blood comes out in a pumping fashion, in time with the heartbeat, and is bright red, then it is from an *artery*. The bleeding must be stopped or the cat will die.

For arteries, if the wound is on the limbs, make a tourniquet by wrapping a bandage, handkerchief, or necktie around the limb, *above* the injury, and inserting a pencil or screwdriver into the bandage, on the side of the wound nearest the heart. Then tighten the tourniquet by twisting the pencil or screwdriver until the bleeding stops.

Blood flowing from a *vein* flows regularly, as opposed to being pumped, and is dark red in color. If the blood is coming from a vein, apply the tourniquet *below* the wound.

It's important to remember that a tourniquet should be just tight enough to stop the bleeding. Loosen the tourniquet every ten minutes to allow the blood to get to the tissues.

Bleeding, emergencies: Unfortunately, there is usually such a bloody mess that you cannot always determine whether the blood is flowing or pumping. Often the wounds are on a part of the body where a tourniquet cannot be applied. So, unless the source of blood is obvious and easily tied off, the best thing you can do is the fastest thing you can do. Grab anything—bandages, a torn shirt, a handkerchief, even a package of tissues—and press over the wound, holding it there as firmly as you can.

Internal bleeding: If the bleeding is internal, or the blood is flowing from the cat's nose or anus, keep the animal still and get it to the vet immediately. (Try not to have another accident while you are rushing to the vet.) Further attempts at first aid will almost certainly do more harm than good. Broken or fractured bones need expert treatment. Leave the job to a professional.

Bandaging

Bandages are used to: stop bleeding; support injured legs; prevent the cat from biting at its injuries; reduce swelling; prevent bacteria from entering the wound and causing infection.

Preferred type of bandage: The easiest type of bandage to use is the Ace ® bandage, available in twelve- and fifteen-foot lengths and in a variety of widths. For bandaging cats, the most useful is the two- or three-inch width. For wounds on the trunk of the cat the four-inch bandage is suggested.

Bandaging the Eye

Technique: Place a moist gauze pad over the affected eye. Wind the bandage around the animal's head, leaving the

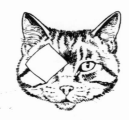

ears in their normal position. Extend the bandage forward

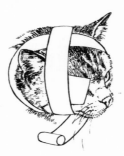

to cover the gauze dressing over the affected eye. Anchor

the bandage with a strip of two- or three-inch adhesive tape

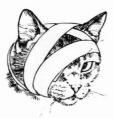

placed at the top of the cat's head. Take care not to wind

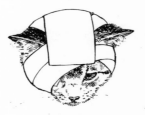

the bandage too tightly, and make sure it does not interfere with the cat's breathing.

Bandaging the Leg

Technique: When bandaging the leg you should bandage the foot as well, to prevent swelling and tissue damage. Pack the spaces between the cat's toes with small wads of cotton to prevent damage to the toes. Wrap cotton

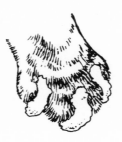

around the foot. Begin bandaging at the top of the leg, go

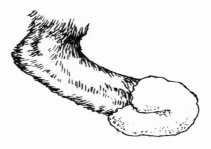

down the front of the leg, around the foot and up the back.

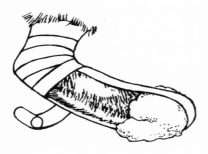

Then wind the bandage around the leg, so that each layer of bandage overlaps the preceding layer, until the whole leg is covered. Tie off the bandage.

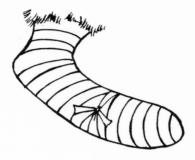

The bandage should be wound firmly enough not to slip, but not so tightly that it stops the circulation. If it is a pressure bandage, intended to stop a hemorrhage, it should be checked every thirty minutes until the bleeding stops.

Cat Up a Tree

A cat sitting on a branch twenty feet off the ground meowing piteously is perhaps a classic example of a potential first aid hazard. It is not, of course, the cat that is in danger but rather the anxious cat lover who tries too hard to rescue kitty.

What to do: If a dog has chased the cat up the tree, chase the dog away. Get a can of cat food or some fish and place it at the foot of the tree. Go home and relax, secure in the knowledge that sooner or later the cat will come down. It will come down the same way it went up. Even if it seems impossible to you, rest assured the cat will manage to climb down somehow. After all, have you ever seen a dead cat in a tree?

Clipping Nails

Cats that do not get enough exercise may need their claws trimmed. If the claws are long enough to catch on fabric, it is time to trim or chance a broken claw.

Technique: Special cat claw clippers are available at

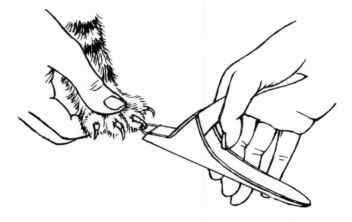

pet stores. If the quick cannot be seen, cut along the line formed by the base of the nail.

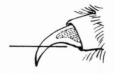

Warning: Do not clip the nail too short or you will cut

the vein under the nail and cause the toe to bleed. Should this happen, the bleeding can be controlled by bandaging the nail (see Bandaging), or by applying a styptic pencil to the site of the bleeding.

Compresses—Hot and Cold

A compress is made by taking a wad of cotton or cotton fabric and saturating it in the proper solution. Cold compresses or ice packs are applied directly over a swelling caused by concussion and will reduce the swelling. Hot compresses are especially effective for reducing pain. They are made by placing the cotton in the hottest water your hands can bear. Wring out the excess water and apply the compress to the affected area for about two minutes. Repeat as often as possible.

Hot and cold compresses may be used together (e.g., for sprains and strains, alternate hot and cold compresses).

Cough Medicines

Cough medicines are designed to soothe or suppress a cough. Before administering cough medicine or soothing syrups, remember that a cough is not a separate entity, but a possible symptom of many diseases. A cough medicine may stop the cough temporarily and allow the cat a rest, but it will not *cure* whatever is causing the cough. If possible, try to determine the cause of the cough before administering the medicine.

Treatment: Administer one 5-mg. tablet of diphenhydramine hydrochloride twice a day (e.g., Benadryl ® or

Hydryllin ®.) To soothe the cat's irritated throat, try a homemade solution of 2 tablespoons of honey and 1 teaspoon lemon juice in 2 tablespoons of water. (See How to Administer Tablets and Pills; Force-Feeding.) If the animal is still coughing after forty-eight hours, consult a vet.

Destruction

Animals in their natural wild state rarely die of old age. Having extended the life span of our cats by protecting them insofar as possible from illness and accident, we have the responsibility of caring for them in their old age and, finally, of sparing them any unnecessary suffering. A part of that responsibility is deciding when that point of unnecessary suffering has been reached. Chronic illness, incontinence, and senility are factors to be balanced against such subjective feelings as the cat owner's love of his pet and the sanctity of life in general.

Although the final decision is the individual cat owner's responsibility, all too often people permit a pet to linger on painfully, hoping that the poor old thing will die soon. When you find yourself feeling that way, perhaps it is time to do your cat one last kindness. When a cat is put to sleep by a veterinarian the process is simple and painless. The cat is given an injection of an anesthetic. Before you can count to three, the cat is dead. Its troubles, aches, and pains are over.

The most difficult situations arise when a cat has been badly injured, usually in an automobile accident, and is in great pain. Most people are not equipped to destroy the animal. So, rather than take the chance of causing even greater pain, call the police at once. They will give you the emergency telephone number of the nearest vet. Leave this sad job to him.

Diet

An adequate diet is one which is palatable and which, when fed regularly, will maintain good health without the development of deficiency diseases. However, some cat owners tend to feed their pet what the animal prefers, or to feed them foods which are convenient to give and/or easy to prepare, without regard for the animal's nutritional requirements. Most cats are accommodating animals: they will eat whatever you give them and will maintain a reasonable nutritional level.

This does not mean that cats can be fed whatever is convenient. Convenience is fine, but a well-balanced diet is essential. A well-balanced diet should contain the correct proportion of proteins, carbohydrates, fats, minerals, and vitamins.

The simplest adequate ration for a healthy cat would consist of good quality raw meat containing about 10 to 20 percent fat, with the occasional addition of offal in the form of heart, liver, or kidneys. Cooked, boned fish can be substituted for meat occasionally.

Canned foods provide a convenient and totally balanced diet, but in some cases the price may be considered prohibitive. We do not recommend the feeding of dried or soft-moist foods exclusively.

Feeding amounts: Four ounces per 10 pounds body weight per day. This figure is based on the assumption that the cat is getting enough exercise. If, for some reason, this is not the case, the food supply should be reduced proportionately, up to half the normal amount.

Special diets: See Orphan Kittens; Diet for Brood Queen; Milk Fever; Nursing Sick Young Cats: Birth to Six Months; Nursing Elderly Cats; Chronic Interstitial Nephritis.

Elizabethan Collar

A most useful device when treating cuts, skin diseases, etc. An Elizabethan collar is a device used to prevent a cat from scratching at its face, ears, or eyes, or from biting various parts of its anatomy. Classically, these collars are prepared from stiff cardboard, but the cat may scratch it apart. We recommend plastic containers (e.g., a small plastic flower pot or child's bucket).

Cut the bottom out of the bucket to a size that the animal's head will go through, punch four more holes around this one, put strings through, and tie it to the cat's collar or around its neck.

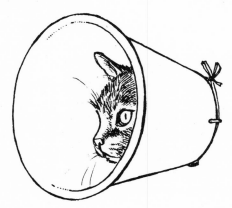

The open end must be far enough away from the nose to prevent licking, and this may present difficulties at feeding time. If so, the collar can be removed briefly to allow eating and drinking. At first, the cat will probably be very distressed by the collar, but this will pass. While your pet will never learn to love the collar, it will learn to live with it.

Emetics (Induced Vomiting)

An emetic is any substance that induces vomiting, and is usually given after a cat has eaten something poisonous. Table salt is a suitable emetic for cats.

Technique: Take a teaspoonful of dry table salt crystals and throw them as far back down the animal's throat as possible. (See How to Open a Cat's Mouth.)

To be effective, the emetic must be administered as soon as possible after the cat has eaten the poison. If the poison has been consumed more than an hour previously, or if the cat is shocked or drowsy, do not induce vomiting.

Warning: Never attempt to make an unconscious animal vomit.

Enema

A enema is an injection of nonirritant fluid into the large intestine, administered by way of the anal passage. The purpose of giving an enema is to empty the large intestine of any abnormal or impacted contents, so that the cat can have a normal bowel movement.

When required: When the cat is constipated. Enemas may be necessary after the consumption of large amounts of bones (not recommended feeding); or particularly with long-haired cats, after they have been licking their coats and have swallowed large amounts of hair.

How to prepare an enema: The best enema solution is produced by lathering some good quality soap into a dish-pan of warm water (¼ pint of warm water with good quality hand soap or soap flakes that contain no detergents or hexachlorophene). This solution is then administered into the rectum via the anus by means of an enema bag. If a ready-made enema is not available, you can improvise, using a length of rubber tubing (approximately one-third inch in diameter) leading to a funnel or a container (e.g., a plastic dishpan with a hole punched in it) filled with the enema solution.

Technique: Spread some newspapers around the area before you give the enema. You will not have time after-wards. Have someone hold the cat. Enemas should only be given with the animal standing. (See Restraint and Han-dling.) Introduce about two inches of tubing into the cat's rectum. A little Vaseline ® on the end of the tubing helps. Hold the container higher than the cat.

Dosage: Administer 1–3 tablespoons of the enema fluid. If the substances that are causing the impaction have not been passed after three attempts, professional help should be sought.

Feeding Times

Cats should be fed regularly at the same hour every day. In this respect, they are creatures of habit: at the accustomed hour, their gastric juices begin to flow.

Kittens: Kittens should receive meals as follows: at eight weeks, feed four times a day; fourteen weeks, three times a day; eighteen weeks, twice a day; six months, one meal a day.

Adult cats: Grown cats may be fed once or twice a day, depending upon the cat's appetite and exercise. Elderly cats should be fed two or even three small meals, rather than one large meal.

First Aid Kit

All cat owners should prepare a first aid kit and keep it in a clearly marked container in a safe place. It should contain:

A pair of sharp-edged, blunt-pointed scissors.
A pair of tweezers.
Four rolls of two-inch adhesive tape.
Four rolls of two-inch Ace ® bandage.
A package of absorbent cotton.
A package of gauze.
A bottle of antiseptic, e.g., hydrogen peroxide.
A razor blade.
A package of needles.
Tylenol ® tablets.
A package of cotton swabs.
Milk of magnesia.

Table salt.
An eyedropper.
A copy of this book.
The vet's address and phone number.

Force-Feeding

When it is necessary to force a cat to eat or drink something, the technique is similar to the one used for the administration of tablets and pills.

Hold the cat: Have an assistant hold the cat while you do the feeding. The assistant holds the cat by the scruff with one hand and wraps his other arm around the animal's back legs. Alternatively, the cat is wrapped in a thick towel or blanket, with only its head protruding. The assistant holds the well-wrapped cat tightly.

Open the cat's mouth: Open the cat's mouth by placing your left hand on top of the animal's head, with your thumb and index finger placed behind the canine teeth (the fangs). Then firmly pull the cat's head backward. This will force the mouth open.

Feeding liquids: The food or fluid is administered with the right hand. Use a plastic spoon if it is a fluid; if the cat does bite down hard, it won't damage its teeth on metal. With the spoon held in your right hand, slowly pour the liquid as far back in the cat's mouth as possible. The slower you pour the contents of the spoon down the cat's throat, the less chance there is of the cat gagging or choking.

Feeding solids: Break the solid food into small, pill-sized bits. Using your right hand, place these bits, one at a time, at the back of the cat's throat. After each bit, hold the cat's head back until the animal licks its nose. This means the cat has swallowed. Open its mouth and feed it another bit.

Flavored meat extracts may be fed simply by rubbing some on the cat's nose. (See Nursing: *Diet.*) A cat will lick anything off its nose. This is often a way of stimulating a sluggish appetite. Once a cat gets a taste off its nose, it may begin to eat voluntarily.

Without assistance: There are easier things than attempting to hold *and* feed a cat on your own. But if you must, get everything ready before you begin. Then use your left hand to open the jaws and your right hand for spooning in whatever it is you are force-feeding. Some cat owners can manage this simply by approaching the animal from behind, squatting down, and holding the cat between their legs while they get on with the job. Other owners who try to force-feed without an assistant have to wrap the cat in a towel, with just its head protruding, and hold the cat by tucking it under their arm. Still others never manage it at all. (It depends to a large extent upon the cat.)

Glucose (Dextrose Monohydrate)

A quick energy source, to be given when the animal is weak and apathetic (available from drugstores). Mix 2–3 tablespoons of dextrose monohydrate with 1 pint of water, or with food.

Substitute: If dextrose monohydrate is not available, add 2 tablespoons of sugar to 1 pint of water; stir until the sugar has dissolved.

Grooming

Most cats will groom themselves, but the wise cat owner does not leave the job entirely to the animal. The act of grooming not only helps the cat keep clean, it also establishes a physical rapport between cat and owner. This rapport will stand the owner in good stead on those occasions when it is necessary to handle the cat in order to administer first aid.

Healthy cats will do their best to keep their coats clean, but even the most industrious cat is unable to keep up with the accumulation of grime in its city environment. It is well to remember that our cats live in a world six inches to two feet in height, about level with automobile exhaust pipes. If the cat's grooming is neglected, and its coat is allowed to become filthy and matted, the cat will develop a predisposition for skin diseases.

Grooming sick animals: The importance of grooming as a factor in nursing, contributing to the cat's well-being, cannot be overemphasized. Sick cats may neglect their grooming; they have an excuse, their owners do not. Apart from the fur, keep the eyes, nose, ears, and the area around the mouth clean by wiping them regularly with a little diluted pHisoDerm ® on cotton: 1 teaspoon of solution to 4 teaspoons of water. A cat with diarrhea will also develop a sore anus. Treat this soreness by applying Vaseline ® or cold cream to the irritated area.

Cats resist water most strenuously and, except in special situations, need not be bathed in water. There are several "dry bath" preparations which will do as well. These are in the form of powder which is dusted into the cat's fur and then brushed out.

All cats should be brushed daily. Long-haired cats should also be combed; any knots of tangled fur that do not comb out should be cut out with scissors. Cats that are not brushed regularly develop hair balls in their stomachs from the accumulation of loose hairs they swallow while grooming themselves. (See Hair Balls.)

How to Administer Tablets and Pills

Concealment: If the cat is not being starved, conceal the pill or tablet in a tasty tidbit (e.g., meat, cheese, or fish). Cats are notorious for finding even the most cunningly concealed pill, so be prepared to administer the pill directly.

Direct technique: Ideally, you should have an assistant. The assistant holds the cat, one hand on the scruff, the other arm wrapped around the cat's back legs. Place your left

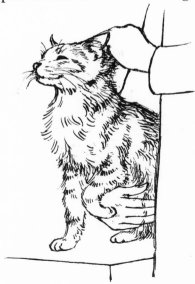

hand on top of the animal's head, with your thumb and index finger placed behind the canine teeth. Pull the cat's

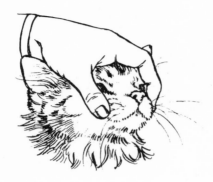

head backward. The tablet is in your right hand. Use this hand to open the cat's mouth by holding the lower jaw behind the lower canine teeth. Place the tablet at the back

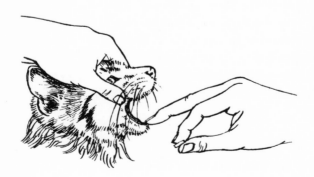

of the cat's throat. Hold the cat's head back, until the animal

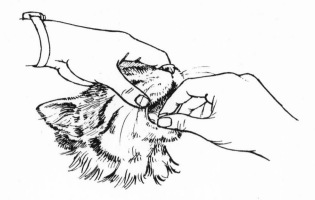

licks its nose. When this happens, the cat has swallowed the tablet.

Unruly cats: Wrap in a blanket or towel, with only the head showing. Slip a loop of bandage behind the lower canine teeth in order to pull the lower jaw down. The upper jaw is held by hand behind the upper canine teeth, as described above. Your assistant administers the tablet by placing it at the back of the cat's throat. Alternatively, a tablet may be crushed between two tablespoons and the powder thrown to the back of the throat. This method is recommended only in especially difficult cases: it may cause increased salivation, which works against the pill's going down and is very likely to bring the pill back up again.

How to Give an Injection

While it is not usual for cat owners to administer injections, there are occasional situations (e.g., in diabetes or certain long courses of antibiotic treatment) when knowledge of the technique can be very useful.

The subcutaneous injection is an injection under the skin; the intravenous injection is an injection directly into the vein. Subcutaneous injections are relatively simple to administer and, when properly given, are completely painless. (Medications requiring intravenous injections are beyond the scope of home treatment.) Be confident and self-assured when giving an injection. If you are hesitant, the cat will sense it and the process will be that much more difficult.

Technique: If there is someone available, ask him to hold your cat for you. (See Restraint and Handling.) Hold the cat firmly by the scruff of the neck. (Some cat owners

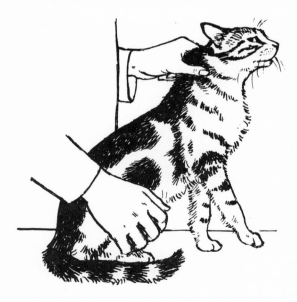

feel that gloves and a heavy coat are useful safety measures, but if the cat is properly scruffed and restrained, they are unnecessary encumbrances.) Saturate a cotton pad with alcohol and swab the skin around the scruff of the neck, where the injection will be administered. Do not make a

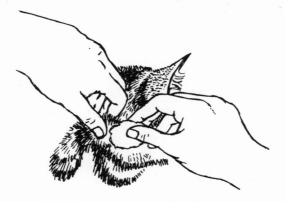

great production of this, or you will alarm the cat. A quick rub with the cotton pad is sufficient. After filling the syringe, hold it point uppermost and slowly press the plunger until all the air is out of the syringe. Hold the syringe at the

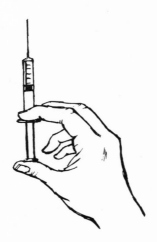

base, between your index finger and thumb. With your other hand, lift a fold of skin at the scruff of the neck into a cone, and slip the needle under the skin below the cone. Press the plunger. Keep the needle as nearly parallel with the skin surface as possible. When the contents of the sy-

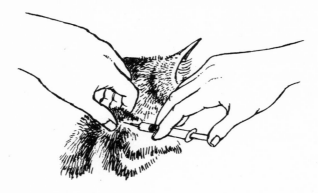

ringe have been injected, withdraw the syringe and rub the site of the injection for a few seconds to make certain the fluid has been dispersed.

If an assistant is not available, you can easily hold most animals by the scruff of the neck with one hand while you administer the injection with the other. In holding the animal by the scruff, you also minimize the danger of being bitten.

How to Open a Cat's Mouth

Technique: To put it mildly, cats can be very difficult about having their mouths opened. If it must be done, here are two ways to accomplish it.

With assistant: Ideally, you should have an assistant who holds the cat while you approach from behind. Then (assuming you are right-handed) place your left hand on top of the cat's head, and the thumb and index finger behind the upper canines (fangs), a finger on each side. Place the remaining fingers of the left hand behind the animal's ears and pivot its head backward. At the same time, open its jaw with your right hand.

Without assistant: If no assistant is available, wrap the cat in a large, thick towel, so that only its head protrudes. Place your thumb and index finger behind the upper canines and the remaining fingers behind the cat's ears. Pivot

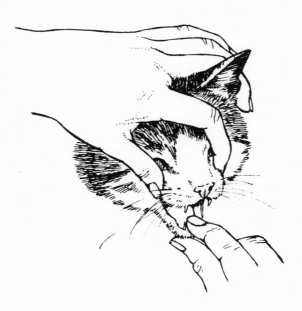

the head backward, and apply slight pressure with your thumb and index finger. This will force the cat to open its mouth. The procedure should be carried out in a calm but determined manner. The secret is to know exactly what you are going to do before you start to do it.

How to Shampoo a Cat

In those extreme instances when it is essential to shampoo a cat, the amount of difficulty experienced depends primarily upon the cat. Some cats will cooperate, others will not. A cat that is accustomed to being handled and groomed is more likely to permit a shampoo without too much fuss.

Difficult cats require an assistant. Have the assistant scruff the cat while you do the shampooing. (See Restraint and Handling.) Be careful not to get soap into the animal's eyes, or it will be twice as difficult next time you shampoo the cat.

If there is no one to help you, put the cat into a pillow-case with its head protruding and wash it through the pillow-case.

Nursing: General Care of Sick Cats

If your pet is suffering from a severe or debilitating disease and is too weak and too sick to groom and feed itself, the nursing and loving care it receives from you will have a vital effect upon its recovery. This nursing care extends to grooming and hygiene as well as to proper feeding. Keep your sick pet clean. Special care should be taken if it is suffering from diarrhea or vomiting, for psychological as well as sanitary reasons. All cats are fastidious and become distressed if allowed to foul themselves. If this occurs, gently wash the animal with soap and water. A dusting of talcum powder after washing is helpful. Apart from doing what is necessary for its well-being, leave a sick cat alone as much as possible. There is a difference between loving care and fussing. Do not fuss over a sick cat.

Diet: A sick cat or one recuperating from an illness needs nourishing food even if the animal does not always want it. Supplement the cat's diet with a mixture of 4 tablespoons of dextrose monohydrate (available from drugstores) to 1 pint of water, daily, to supply extra energy. Serve the mixture in place of the cat's regular drinking water. Do not give this or any fluids to a cat that is vomiting. (See Excessive Thirst.) If the cat does have an appetite, do not give it all it wants at one time. Feed it small amounts at frequent intervals.

If the cat has no appetite, try to tempt it with strong-smelling foods (e.g., cheese, chicken livers, fish, canned sardines). A cat's sense of smell, if properly enticed, will often start it eating again. Homemade meat extracts often do the trick. These are made by mincing raw meat as finely as possible and pouring boiling water over it. The resulting liquid is then poured into a bowl, and a pinch of salt and a tiny pinch of monosodium glutamate are added to bring out the flavor.

Make every effort to tempt the cat voluntarily. As a last resort, you will have to force-feed. Remember that the smallest amount of food taken voluntarily will do more good than a much larger amount that has been force-fed. (See Force-Feeding.)

Hygiene: Scrupulous hygiene is absolutely essential to successful nursing. Therefore, all bowls, dishes, spoons, etc., that come in contact with the cat must be sterilized in boiling water after each meal.

Nursing Elderly Cats

Elderly cats present special problems, and their general condition can be greatly improved by feeding them good quality foods in proper amounts.

When nursing an older cat whose appetite is sluggish, stimulate the appetite by feeding meat extracts and flavorings. Since a cat's sense of smell and taste diminish with age, extra attention to diet is necessary to keep the sick elderly cat eating. Remember, cats will not eat food that they cannot smell.

Most elderly cats are nephritic (i.e., they suffer from kidney problems), and should be fed a diet composed of white meat (fish or chicken) and carbohydrates, in the form of rice or hominy grits, mixed into their food. Some cats dislike rice or grits. Faced with this, the best solution is to put the rice into a blender and mix it very well with some food that they do like. Special therapeutic diets are also available from the veterinarian.

Elderly cats should be given all the water they can drink. Be sure the cat's drinking bowl is always full. Supplement the cat's diet with vitamin A and vitamin B_{12} tablets.

Nursing Sick Young Cats: Birth to Six Months

Diet is of paramount importance in the successful nursing of young cats. When cats develop infections, their food intake falls. This is particularly dangerous in kittens, who are very dependent upon daily nutrition. When young cats stop eating, they set in motion a cycle of malnutrition and further infection that ultimately ends in death. A cat weighing 2 pounds requires at least 8 teaspoons of water daily. It also needs minerals, protein, carbohydrates, fats, and vitamins. (See Diet.)

If there is no diarrhea or vomiting, add powdered cow's milk to the kitten's diet, at twice the strength recommended for human babies. For orphan kittens, milk substitutes of the kind used in feeding babies are a complete diet. Feed every two hours for the first week, day and night; afterwards, every three hours for ten days.

If there is diarrhea or vomiting, neither milk nor milk products should be given. Withhold all food for twelve hours, then feed a mixture of ½ pint water, 3 tablespoons dextrose monohydrate, 1 raw egg white, and a pinch of salt. Small portions of deboned chicken or fish may be given three or four times a day for four days.

If the kitten still refuses to eat after twenty-four hours, consult a vet. If a vet is not available, force-feed with a meat extract until food is taken voluntarily. (See Nursing: General, *Diet.*) Continue the water and dextrose monohydrate mixture as well, force-feeding if necessary. (See Force-Feeding; Orphan Kittens.)

Orphan Kittens

Very young kittens (up to four weeks old) without a mother, or those from a mother unable to breast-feed them (see Agalactia), should be placed in a small, warm box and fed a substitute milk supplement every two hours for the first two weeks (day and night). After that they should be fed every three hours. (See *Feeding technique* below.)

After each feeding the kittens should be burped: rub the

abdomen and genitals gently with an oiled finger so as not to irritate their tender skin. The burping is normally accompanied by urination and defecation.

Homemade milk supplement: If commercial substitutes are not available, you can make your own milk supplement. Combine: 30 ounces of cow's milk, 1 egg yolk, a pinch of bone meal, a pinch of citric acid. Stir the mixture and keep it in the refrigerator. Warm it to 100°F. before feeding.

Feeding technique: Use an eyedropper or doll's feeding bottle. Be sure to clean thoroughly and boil the dropper or doll's bottle after each feeding. The amount of food required will vary with the size of the kittens. Generally, they should be fed according to their appetite. Unfortunately, some kittens have appetites larger than their capacity.

Diarrhea: Overfeeding may result in diarrhea. Should diarrhea develop, withhold milk supplement and give the kitten lukewarm boiled water with dextrose monohydrate added (3 tablespoons of dextrose monohydrate to 1 pint of water) for two feedings. If the diarrhea stops, return to the milk supplement. If the diarrhea persists for longer than twenty-four hours, call the vet. If the diarrhea was not caused by overfeeding, it may be the result of an infection.

Solid foods: After three weeks of age, kittens will show an interest in more adult food. Encourage this new appetite by feeding them bits of deboned chicken and fish, and minced meat. If these delicacies are not available, substitute canned or dry cat food.

Weaning: Taking young animals off their mother's milk, or off the milk supplement, should be completed by the time the kittens are four to six weeks old.

Poultices

The application of heat to a swelling or to a sore area will relieve the pain and control the swelling. The advantage of a poultice is that it retains heat without having to be changed constantly.

There are several types of poultices; the simplest and one of the most effective is a kaolin poultice. (Kaolin is a fine, white china clay, sometimes called "heavy kaolin," available in cans from most pharmacies.)

Prepare the poultice by heating a can of kaolin in a saucepan of boiling water. When the clay is fairly hot, spread it on a bandage, and tape it over the affected area. Before placing the bandage on the cat, test a bit of the kaolin on the back of your hand. It should be very warm, but not hot enough to cause any pain. The poultice should be changed every four hours.

Substitutes: If kaolin is not available, a poultice may be made from bread or potatoes. To make a poultice from bread, boil some water and soak a piece of bread in it. Allow it to cool enough for you to handle it, then apply it to a bandage and tape the bandage over the affected area. To make a poultice from potatoes, mash some freshly cooked potatoes and apply them to a bandage. Tape the bandage over the affected area.

Restraint and Handling

By restraint we mean the technique of handling, moving, and holding a cat, usually against its will. (See also How to Open a Cat's Mouth; How to Shampoo a Cat; How to Administer Tablets and Pills.)

When to use restraint: When one must do something which the cat finds frightening, painful, or objectionable. It. is never pleasant to use restraint, but when it is necessary, be firm and unhurried. The trick is to know what you are going to do *before* you approach your cat. There are several methods of restraining reluctant animals. The method you choose depends upon the temperament of the cat and your purpose in restraining the cat. That is, do you want to move the animal, or to hold it?

Techniques: Difficult cats may be captured by throwing a coat or blanket over them and handling them through it. Docile cats may be scruffed. To scruff a cat, take a firm grip with one hand on the loose flesh just behind the cat's head. Hold tight enough so that the cat cannot turn its head, but not so tightly that it is in pain (see illustration on page 40 for scruffing cat). Wrap the cat in a towel, with its head protruding. This is the best way of holding a cat without an assistant.

Saline Solution

A sterile (germ-free) salt solution. Dissolve 1 teaspoon of iodine-free table salt in 1 pint of boiling water. Allow the water to cool to body temperature before applying.

Taking the Pulse

Technique: Place your index finger and forefinger over the cat's femoral artery at the point where it crosses the thigh bone on the inside of the thigh, almost in the groin.

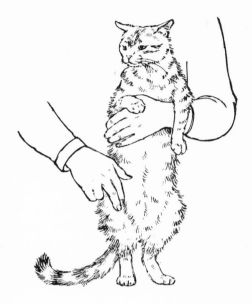

Count the pulse beats for ten seconds and multiply by six.

Normally, the pulse rate varies from 110–140 beats a minute when the cat is in good health. The cat owner should always know his pet's normal pulse rate, so that a higher or lower rate will not go unnoticed. A very slow pulse, 30–50 beats a minute, indicates that the cat is very ill and requires immediate professional treatment. A very low pulse rate appears in cases of sedative overdose and in the final, declining stages of infection. In a cat that is running a fever, there will be a persistent high pulse rate, as rapid as 160 beats a minute. This condition also demands immediate professional treatment.

Taking Samples of Feces and Urine

Technique: To assist the vet in diagnosing certain illnesses, a specimen of the cat's feces or urine will be needed. Since cats do not always perform at the most convenient time and place, this may require some persistence on the owner's part. To collect urine from the cat, put a few spoonfuls of sand or kitty litter in a tray, and prop up one end of the tray so that the urine flows to the other end. Be careful not to put in so much sand that it absorbs all the urine. If your cat goes outdoors, the secret of collecting a sample of feces or urine is to keep the cat indoors until it has delivered.

Collect the urine (a few drops will suffice) or feces immediately and put it in a can or bottle clearly labeled with the cat's name, the owner's name, and the date.

Taking Temperature

Most infectious and contagious diseases in the early stages cause the body temperature to rise. This rise is often, but not always, accompanied by lethargy and loss of appetite. Identification of fever and its severity provides the cat owner with a guide as to whether the vet should be consulted.

Contrary to uninformed opinion, taking a cat's temperature is not at all difficult. The technique is simple.

Type of thermometer: Any stubby, bulbed clinical thermometer may be used. Such thermometers are available at drugstores.

Technique: A cat's temperature must always be taken rectally. (If you put a thermometer in the cat's mouth, it will probably try to eat it.) Have someone hold the cat while you take its temperature. (See Restraint and Handling.) A well-trained pet should allow its owner to take its temperature without making too much of a fuss. Hold the thermometer by the end opposite the bulb between your thumb and index finger; shake it with a sharp, jerky movement until the mercury is down to 95°F. On your first try, it is best to do this over a thick rug or bed (if you do drop the thermometer, it will not break). Dip the bulb of the thermometer in Vaseline ® or cold cream. Approach the cat from the rear, and gently slide one inch of the thermometer through the anal sphincter, using a gentle rotary action. Be prepared to stop the cat from trying to sit down. Cats are very conscious of their anal sphincters and unless great care is taken the cat may react violently and you may break the thermometer. So work the thermometer in slowly and gently. (If the thermometer breaks, take the cat to a vet immediately. If a vet is not available, administer mineral oil, 1 tablespoon orally three times a day, until the thermometer is expelled with feces.)

Push the thermometer in with a light touch, letting it find its own direction. Once the thermometer is in place, support the protruding end very lightly and wait one full minute. Withdraw the thermometer, wipe it clean with cotton or tissue, and read the temperature. Normal body temperature in cats is 101°F. A temperature of 102.5°F. or higher is a good reason to consult a vet.

When calculating temperatures, remember that an excited or frightened animal has a higher body temperature than a relaxed animal. Subtract a degree or two if this is the case. When you have finished using the thermometer, wash it in *cold* water and sterilize by dipping it into alcohol.

Teeth Care

Cats should have regular dental checkups by a veterinarian, to prevent gingivitis, periodontitis, halitosis, and eventual tooth loss. The wise owner will clean the cat's teeth regularly from an early age with toothpaste or a mild, abrasive cleaning powder on cotton. If the owner accustoms the cat to having its teeth cleaned while it is still very young, the animal will remain cooperative when it is grown.

Tourniquets

The purpose of a tourniquet is to cut off the flow of blood pumping from the heart out through a severed artery or vein.

In an emergency, a tourniquet can be improvised; a necktie, a belt, a strip of material, a shoelace, even a strip of plaited grass will serve. If the cat is bleeding badly, try to stanch the bleeding to observe the way the blood is flowing. This indicates whether the cat is bleeding from an artery or a vein.

Arterial wounds: Blood that comes out in a pumping fashion, in time with the heartbeat, and is bright red, is from an artery; the bleeding must be stopped quickly or the cat will die.

Treatment: For arterial wounds (on the limbs), make a tourniquet by wrapping the bandage or belt around the limb, above the injury. Insert a pencil or screwdriver into

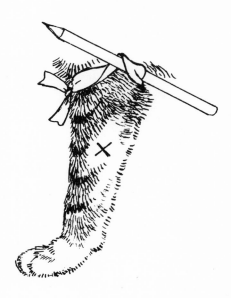

the bandage, on the side of the wound nearest the heart. Twist the tourniquet until the bleeding stops.

Venous wounds: Blood flowing from a vein flows regularly, rather than being pumped out; the color is dark red.

Treatment: For venous wounds, apply the tourniquet below the wound and twist it until the bleeding stops.

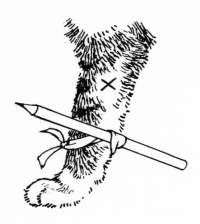

Note: Keep the tourniquet tight for not more than one minute. Then loosen it slightly. Loosen the tourniquet completely every ten minutes to see whether the bleeding has stopped and to allow the blood to reach the rest of the leg and prevent tissue damage.

Transportation of Injured Cats

If an injured cat must be moved, before you do anything, know exactly what you are going to do and where you are going to move it. A little forethought can save a great deal of agony. Remember, a cat in pain will attempt to bite and scratch. Be careful when you approach the cat. (See Restraint and Handling.)

Before you move an injured cat: If the cat is bleeding profusely, stop the bleeding. Check for a possible *fractured spine* by pinching the injured cat's toes. If the animal does not register pain, there is a possibility that the spine is fractured. In this event, do not move the cat unless it is absolutely essential.

Technique for moving an injured cat: A cat may be lifted by the scruff of the neck and carried to your car. If there is someone with you, have him hold the injured animal while you drive. If you are alone, place the cat on the floor of the car, in the front, on the passenger side.

Serious injuries may require a sling of some sort. Wrap the cat in a coat or a blanket and place it on the floor of the car. If a stretcher is used, roll, do not lift, the cat onto it. Cover the injured cat with a blanket or coat. This will help to minimize the danger of shock, by keeping the animal warm as well as providing a degree of restraint. Do not give the injured cat anything to drink, no water, no alcohol. This is to prevent vomiting if an anesthetic has to be administered.

Vaccination

Definition: A vaccine is an injection of a preparation of living or dead viruses that stimulates the formation of immunity to certain viral or bacterial diseases.

Natural immunity: Kittens receive antibodies from the mother's first milk (colostrum). This provides a natural immunity that lasts for eight to ten weeks and then diminishes. In order not to interfere with this natural immunity, kittens are usually not vaccinated until they are eight weeks old.

Orphans: Orphan kittens, which are being fed on supplement and have not received colostrum, should be vaccinated at eight weeks and again at twelve weeks of age to insure a high immunity.

Cat vaccines: Cats should be vaccinated at eight weeks of age to prevent infections of feline enteritis. This should be repeated in two weeks, with boosters annually.

Weaning

Weaning is the process of taking a kitten off its mother's milk and putting it on a diet of more adult foods. Kittens begin showing an interest in solid foods at three or four weeks of age. This does not mean that they are quite ready to be weaned. But their interest should be encouraged by offering them small amounts of finely chopped meat, deboned fish or chicken, and bowls of milk three or four times a day.

When the kittens are five to six weeks old they are ready to be weaned. At this time the mother begins to vomit her food (soft, partially digested) for her youngsters to eat. At about eight weeks of age, recently weaned kittens should be fed five meals a day.

2

Problems of the Head and Neck

THE EAR

Acute Middle Ear Infection

Cause: Usually seen as the result of simple ear complaints that have been left untreated.

Symptoms: Loss of balance. The cat may walk around with its head constantly on one side. Sometimes the cat keeps falling over. (See also Unconsciousness; Poisoning.) There may also be deafness and vomiting.

Treatment: These symptoms constitute an emergency. The infection can spread to the brain rapidly, causing severe meningitis, encephalitis, and death. Immediate professional assistance is vital.

Acute Otitis

Symptoms: May be similar to those of ear mites (see Ear Mites), but this bacterial condition produces much inflammation and soreness.

Treatment: Acute otitis cannot be cured at home. Consult a veterinarian. To relieve the acute itching and soreness, pour warm olive oil into the ear. To relieve discomfort, administer one-half of a 250-mg. Tylenol ® tablet to an adult cat, once only. (See How to Administer Tablets and Pills.)

Remember that these are only temporary measures to be used until professional help is available.

Warning: If left untreated, this condition can develop into a middle ear infection.

Bleeding or Hemorrhaging from the Ear

Often seen after fights or road accidents. Bleeding may be from the earflap or from inside the ear.

Treatment: Whether the bleeding originates from the earflap or from the ear itself, the treatment is the same. Pack the ear canal with cotton (just enough to fill the ear) and hold in place.

Warning: If left untreated, this condition can develop into a middle ear infection.

Blood Blister on the Ear (Hematoma)

A thick, fluctuating, irregular swelling usually found inside the earflap, but the outside may be involved as well. The blister itself is painless and firmer than an abscess.

Causes: These blisters arise suddenly, usually as the result of a blow or a bite, an ear mite infection, or from an irritation that causes constant scratching. Such an irritation might be caused by an infection in the ear, and will be accompanied by pus from the ear canal.

Treatment: If the blister is the result of an ear infection and is small, leave it alone and treat the infection. (See Acute Middle Ear Infection.)

Treatment for persistent blister: If the blister has not disappeared after three or four days, minor surgery will be required to drain, curette, and suture it. This should be left to a professional. If the persistent blister is fairly small (approximately one-half inch in diameter), you can drain it yourself. Sterilize a needle by boiling it for twenty minutes, wash your hands, prick the blister on the inside of the earflap with the sterile needle, and allow it to drain naturally. For large blisters, consult a vet.

Hematomas, while not serious in themselves, can easily cause permanent disfigurement of the ear. The best first aid is to keep the ears bandaged and taped to the cat's head to prevent the animal from making them worse. If the cat persists in scratching, use an Elizabethan collar. (See Elizabethan Collar.)

Deafness

Deafness may be either hereditary or acquired.

Hereditary deafness: Usually found in white cats with blue eyes. Cats suffering from hereditary deafness should be sterilized to prevent them from passing on the condition.

Acquired deafness: Acquired deafness often occurs as the result of ear infections or accidents. It may be temporary or irreversible, depending upon the cause and severity of the condition.

Partial deafness: Partial deafness occurs in elderly cats, and in younger ones which have ingested poisons containing lead.

Symptoms: Deaf cats may appear to be stupid, do not respond to their names or to commands, and meow continually. A definite diagnosis of true deafness is difficult, since the deaf cat is compensated by the enhancement of its other sensory perceptions, especially its ability to detect vibrations.

Ear Mites (Otodectic Mange)

Otodectic mange mites are common in cats.

Symptoms: Usually, the first symptom observed is a crumbly, waxy, dark brown discharge containing brown crusts in and around the ears. There is acute irritation of the ears, and the cat spends much time scratching its ears and shaking its head vigorously. There may be a rattling noise from the ears when the cat shakes its head.

Treatment: An assistant is helpful, although not absolutely essential. Wrap the cat in a towel with only its head protruding. Then clean the cat's ears with cotton dipped in a small amount of a very dilute mixture of mild liquid detergent (1 teaspoon of liquid detergent to ½ cup of water). This will get rid of the sticky wax.

Be careful when cleaning the ears, but you need not be afraid of touching the eardrum since it is well out of the way of a pad or ball of cotton. Do not use a cotton swab or Q-tip ®, as this may damage the eardrum.

After cleaning, swab the inside of the ears with olive oil or mineral oil twice a day for three weeks. Use the oil sparingly. Hold the earflaps while applying the solution. This stops the animal from shaking its head. If the condition has not improved after three to four days of home treatment, seek professional help.

Also rub oil into the tail tip, for cats sleep curled up.

Foreign Body in the Ear

Symptoms: Excessive shaking of the head, scratching of the ear.

Treatment: Most foreign bodies in the ear can be removed by pouring a little olive oil or cooking oil into the ear and gentle massaging the ear until the object is floated out. If the foreign body does not float out, contact a veterinarian. The urgency of the case can be gauged by the cat's behavior.

Warning: Do not poke anything smaller than your left elbow into the cat's ear (i.e., do not put *anything* except a small cotton ball into the cat's ear). Never use a swab. (See Acute Otitis.)

THE EYE

Blindness

Sudden blindness: The result of either a stroke or an accident in which the cat's brain or eyes have been injured.

Temporary blindness: This occurs during infections of the clear part of the eye (e.g., keratitis). If not properly treated, these infections can give rise to clouding and, eventually, ulceration of the cornea (corneal ulcer).

If a corneal ulcer occurs, immediate professional treatment is vital. Do not bathe the eye. Corneal ulcers take a long time to heal and the cat may be left with a black scar on the cornea.

Progressive blindness: This common condition is usually the result of old age or the formation of cataracts due to diabetes.

Treatment: If you suspect that your cat is going blind, and the symptoms are painfully obvious (bumping into things, inability to recognize people at a distance), have the cat examined by a vet. He will make a definite diagnosis and may improve the condition by surgery or enzyme injections.

If the condition is irreversible, the cat owner should be aware that blindness need not be the end of the animal's life. When the eyes fail, the cat's other senses develop to compensate. Blind animals, as a rule, have a much better sense of hearing and smell than sighted animals. By the time the cat is completely blind, it will know its way around the house. Blind animals, on the whole, manage remarkably well. They just need a little extra care.

Brown Stains in the Corner of the Eye

Certain cats, especially all-white cats, may develop brown staining in the corners of their eyes.

Cause: Blockage or absence of tear ducts.

Treatment: Prepare a dilute solution of hydrogen peroxide (1 part peroxide to 10 parts water) and bathe the stains liberally. Do not bathe the eyeball, only the stains.

This not only gets rid of the stains, but it may also remove the obstruction in blockage of the tear ducts.

Cataracts

A cataract is an opacity and hardening of the lens of the eye that prevents light from passing through it.

Causes: The most common cause of cataracts is old age. But it must be remembered that cataracts cause varying degrees of blindness. In an elderly cat, the lens may appear quite opaque, yet a certain amount of vision may still be possible. When cataracts appear in the eyes of young cats, a disease (e.g., diabetes) must be considered.

Symptoms: A gradual, growing opacity or cloudiness of the pupil. The cataract itself resembles a white marble inside the eye.

Treatment: Cataracts, like every serious eye condition, must be treated by a professional. This treatment should be started as soon as the cat owner notices the cloudiness. Delay can prevent possible cure. In many cases a nonfunctional lens can be removed surgically, resulting in the return of a fair degree of vision.

Conjunctivitis

Although it is not contagious to humans, conjunctivitis can be transmitted from animal to animal. Quarantine the infected cat.

Symptoms: Painful red eye, sore to the touch; sticky yellowish discharge exuded from the eye; cat continually rubs its face on the ground.

Treatment: Prepare a saline solution: add 1 teaspoon of table salt to 1 pint of boiling water. Allow the solution to cool before using. Bathe the eye liberally with the solution every two hours for the next twenty-four hours. Soak a wad of absorbent cotton in the saline solution and then squeeze the cotton so that the solution floods the eye. If the condition does not clear up within thirty-six hours, seek professional help.

Eyeball Out of Socket

This condition sometimes results from fights or highway accidents.

Treatment: Apply olive oil or Vaseline ® to the eye socket, and gently try to ease the eyeball back into place. Then bandage over. If the eyeball will not stay in the eye socket, hold the eye in with a pad of damp or oily cotton. (Saturate cotton with olive oil.) Bandage lightly. (See Bandaging the Eye.) Seek professional help immediately.

Foreign Body in the Eye

The foreign body may be a grass seed, a bit of grit, or a grain of sand. Anything that does not belong in the eye is called a foreign body.

Symptoms: Sudden and profuse tearing. The tears flow from one eye only. There will be acute irritation of that eyeball as well.

Treatment: Make a sterile saline solution by adding 1 teaspoon of table salt to 1 pint of water. Bring the water to a boil. Allow time for the water to cool. Bathe the eye liberally with cooled saline solution, using an eyedropper, or a saturated wad of cotton squeezed into the eye.

Apply a soothing ophthalmic ointment (your pharmacist can advise you about the brand) directly into the eyeball. Place the thumb and index finger of the left hand above and below the affected eye. Squeeze the ointment into the corner of the eye with your right hand. Close the eyelid with the thumb and index finger of your left hand and hold it closed for a few seconds. This will spread the ointment over the whole eyeball.

If the cat persists in scratching its eye after the treatment you may not have flushed out the object. Take the cat to the vet, and leave further treatment to him.

Do not attempt to remove an object that has punctured the eyeball. In addition to the extreme pain it causes, the object will actually protrude from the eyeball. Seek professional help.

Glaucoma (Swelling of the Eye)

Cause: This condition, though rare in cats, does occur. It is caused by failure of the fluid in the eye to circulate properly, resulting in a rise in pressure inside the eye.

Symptoms: The eyeball increases in size and protrudes from the eye socket. The animal is depressed and irritable. There is associated conjunctivitis and, in later stages, corneal opacity (a milkiness of the eye).

Treatment: Glaucoma *must* be treated by a veterinarian; he will administer drugs to improve the circulation of fluid.

Prolapsed Third Eyelid

In cats this condition indicates a mild illness (e.g., slight nephritis or a case of mild cat flu). The third eyelid comes from the inner corner of the eye and covers the entire eyeball. When this third eyelid is prolapsed, it does not retract normally, but covers a part or all of the eyeball.

Treatment: There is no need to treat the prolapsed eyelid, since it is only a symptom. Treat the cause (i.e., the disease state) by giving the cat an extra supplement of vitamins: one 50-mg. tablet of vitamin B_{12} twice a day, plus one capsule of vitamin A (500 units) per day. Take care not to exceed the vitamin A dosage. (See also How to Administer Tablets and Pills.)

If the cat is eating normally, there is no cause for alarm. But if the third eyelid does not return to normal within three or four days, have the cat examined by a vet.

THE MOUTH

Bad Breath (Halitosis)

Generally, a cat with bad breath is not well. If the condition persists for more than forty-eight hours, seek professional advice.

Causes: In cats under six months of age, bad breath sometimes accompanies teething. It also may indicate a worm infestation. In older cats, bad breath suggests a number of disease states: tonsillitis, stomach infection, stomatitis, stomach ulcer, infected or broken teeth, labial eczema, or sinusitis. In elderly cats, continuing halitosis usually indicates a degree of chronic kidney failure.

Treatment: Check for disease states. Does the cat act sick? Is it feverish? Apathetic? Once these disease states have been eliminated as possible causes, treat the condition by administering chlorophyll or charcoal tablets, one a day. Continue the treatment even after the breath has been cleansed. (See How to Administer Tablets and Pills.)

Broken Tooth

Occasionally, a cat will break a tooth by biting on something harder than its tooth.

Symptoms: Drooling; slight bleeding from the mouth.

Treatment: This is not an emergency, although the broken tooth may have to be extracted eventually. Very cold or very hard substances can further damage the exposed portion of the tooth.

Gingivitis

Gingivitis is an acute or chronic infection of the gums that appears at the margin of the teeth and gums. It is often seen in association with tartar.

Causes: Gingivitis is often caused by general infections of the mouth and throat as well as by more specific infections.

Symptoms: The classic symptom is a narrow red line along the gum, above the tooth or teeth; halitosis; the gums bleed easily.

Treatment: Gingivitis is easily treated by applying a solution made of 1 part hydrogen peroxide to 3 parts water. Swab the gums with this solution every three hours. (See also How to Open a Cat's Mouth.) If the condition has not cleared up after three days of treatment, seek professional help to identify and eliminate the exact cause of the condition.

Specific Abscess: Tooth Root or Molar Abscess

The "specific" abscess is found on the upper tooth roots.

Cause: Decayed tooth.

Symptoms: If an abscess constantly recurs below the cat's eye or along the line of the jaw, examine the cat's mouth. A decayed tooth may be causing the abscess. The abscess itself is a pus-discharging sore that appears on the cat's face. (See abscesses.)

Treatment: There is no home treatment for this condition. Tooth root abscesses require extraction of the tooth and antibiotic treatment. Consult a veterinarian.

Tartar on the Teeth

Causes: All cats living in hard water areas eventually develop tartar on their teeth. Tartar and periodontitis (an infection of the gums) may be related, especially in older animals, to chronic kidney (renal) failure.

Symptoms: Hard, dull brown crusts that spread from the gums across the teeth; bad breath (halitosis); excessive salivation; pawing and rubbing at the mouth. The cat, while obviously hungry, refuses to eat, or begins to eat and spits out the food. The tartar causes pain at the margin of the gums and teeth when the cat chews its food. Should these symptoms occur, examine your cat's teeth.

Treatment: In hard water areas, give the cat boiled or distilled water to drink. With docile cats, during the early stages, tartar can be rubbed off with smoker's tooth powder. Remember, tartar accumulates on both the front and back teeth. In particularly stubborn cases, professional scaling by a vet may be necessary.

Prevention: Prevention of tartar accumulation can be accomplished by regular (once a month) cleaning of the cat's teeth with ordinary toothpaste on cotton or smoker's tooth powder on moist cotton.

Technique for cleaning cat's teeth: Wrap the cat in a towel, with only its head protruding. With the cat tucked under your arm, lift the animal's lips and gently swab the moist cotton over its teeth. It may sound impossible, but most cats don't mind having their teeth cleaned. After the first few times they accept it as part of their regular grooming and, in some instances, may even cooperate. If cotton is difficult to manage, use a child's toothbrush; it affords more leverage.

Teething Stages

Like humans, cats have two sets of teeth. The temporary teeth (baby teeth) appear about three weeks after birth.
These are replaced by the permanent teeth which appear
from five months onward. As the permanent teeth push
through the gums, they displace the temporary teeth,
which are either spit out or swallowed. By six or seven
months of age, all the permanent teeth are in. Adult cats
have twenty-six temporary teeth and thirty permanent
teeth.

THE TONGUE

Bitten Tongue

Symptoms: Profuse bleeding from the mouth.
Treatment: A bitten tongue may sound like a minor
mishap, but if the bleeding is very heavy it is an emergency.
Since the tongue is constantly moist and moving, it is difficult for a blood clot to form, so that bleeding is continuous.
If the cut is deep enough, the cat can bleed to death (it
would take at least twenty-four hours for this to happen). If
the cat will allow it, hold the animal's tongue in a cotton
pad to reduce the bleeding while you are transporting it to
the vet.

Inflammation of the Tongue (Glossitis)

Causes: Numerous; most of them serious. Can be the

result of chronic interstitial nephritis, cat flu, corrosive poisons, wounds, or other trauma.

Symptoms: Severe dribbling; loss of appetite; halitosis. Open the cat's mouth and look for raw, red, sore, circular patches. These are ulcers on the tongue. In the later stages, there is a foul, brownish drainage from the corner of the mouth that drips down the chest and paws. Look for drainage stains on the cat's chest and paws.

Treatment: The cat's mouth must be kept as clean as possible. Wash it out with a dilute solution of hydrogen peroxide (add 1 teaspoon peroxide to 3 teaspoons water). Apply solution every two hours for twenty-four hours. If the inflammation persists after twenty-four hours, seek professional help.

THE NOSE

Nasal Discharge

A thick, yellowish mucus discharge may be a symptom of one of the feline virus diseases. Normally, a healthy cat's nose is cold and wet. A hot, dry nose suggests a fever and illness and warrants further investigation. Consult a veterinarian. (See also Sinusitis.)

Nosebleed (Epistaxis)

Nosebleeds are symptoms. The cat owner should be more concerned with the cause than with the nosebleed itself. In most cases, a nosebleed will subside naturally in a short time.

Causes: Nosebleeds can be the result of: an automobile

accident; tumors; decayed tooth sockets; excessive sneezing; high blood pressure; or foreign bodies or minute parasites in the nose.

Treatment: Sponge the nostrils dry with absorbent cotton. Examine the nostrils under a bright light to determine the cause or site of the hemorrhage. If a foreign body is visible, remove it with tweezers. If you cannot see anything, do not poke about in the cat's nostrils. The mucous membrane that lines the nostrils is very sensitive and easily injured.

If the cause of the nosebleed is not apparent, keep the cat as still as possible. Apply cold compresses or ice cubes to the bridge of the nose. If this treatment does not stop the bleeding, or if the bleeding continues intermittently, get professional assistance. The degree of urgency is determined by the severity of the bleeding.

Tip of the nose: Bleeding from the tip of the nose can be persistent and, if too much blood is lost, potentially dangerous. It can be controlled by pressure with the fingers.

Sinusitis

Sinusitis is an infection of the sinuses—an extension of the nasal chamber, located in the front of the cat's head.

Causes: The infection may be caused either by germs or by a foreign body in the nose.

Symptoms: Yellowish mucous discharge; bouts of sneezing; loss of appetite. Except in the case of foreign bodies, sinusitis rarely occurs on its own. It is usually seen as a sequel to virus conditions (e.g., cat flu).

Treatment: Since many other illnesses are characterized by these same symptoms, you will need professional help to make a correct diagnosis. If the symptoms continue for more than twenty-four hours, take the cat to the vet. (If it is sinusitis, the vet will probably administer a course of antibiotics.)

If a vet is not immediately available, home treatment consists of keeping the cat's face clean of the mucous discharge, and helping the animal to breathe normally by clearing its nasal passages. This is accomplished by having the cat inhale a preparation of menthol crystals (available from drugstores) in hot water. To make this preparation, place some boiling water in a large, shallow tin dish (a pie tin), and add a pinch of menthol crystals. Then, calmly but firmly, hold the cat's face over the steam for a moment or two.

Try to treat this procedure as an ordinary occurrence. The trick is to have the cat inhale as much of the vapor as possible, and this can only be achieved if the cat is not alarmed. Since you do not want to hold a struggling, frightened animal over boiling water, do not force your cat. Handle the animal with confidence.

Sneezing

Continual sneezing is a much more serious symptom in cats than in people.

Intermittent sneezing: If the cat sneezes on and off for a few hours, but seems all right otherwise—no fever, apathy, etc.—the sneezing is probably due to simple irritation (e.g., a bit of dust up its nose).

Prolonged sneezing: If the cat continues to sneeze throughout the day, with accompanying nasal discharge, suspect an infection. Get professional help.

Strenuous sneezing: Strenuous and continued sneezing suggests a foreign body in the nose.

Examine the nostrils with a flashlight. If the foreign object is visible, use tweezers and remove it carefully. If you do not see anything, don't poke about with the tweezers. The nasal lining is easily ruptured. (See Nosebleed.)

THE THROAT

Choking

Choking takes place when either the tongue or a foreign body blocks the back of the throat and prevents the cat from breathing. Choking often looks and sounds much worse than it is because the cat panics, which makes it choke even more, which makes it panic even more. . . . Don't you panic, too!

Treatment: If the cat has fainted (from lack of oxygen), open its mouth and pull its tongue out, making sure that nothing is blocking the windpipe. If there is an obstruction, do not try to push it down the cat's throat. Hook it out with your finger. If the cat is still unconscious once the throat is clear, administer artificial respiration.

If the cat is conscious, hold it upside down by its hind legs and thump it on the back. This may dislodge the object. If it does not, and the cat is still choking, open its mouth (see Restraint and Handling) and use your fingers to fish out the foreign object. If it is stuck, carefully pour a little olive oil down the animal's throat to lubricate the gullet. If your probing causes the cat to gag, so much the better; this may bring the obstruction up and out.

Cats are not very cooperative when it comes to having

their mouths pried open, but if it must be done, here's how. Get an assistant to hold the cat. Approach the head from behind. Then (assuming you are right-handed), place your left hand on top of the cat's head, and your thumb and index finger behind the upper canines (fangs), a finger on each side. Place the remaining fingers behind the animal's ears and pivot its head backward. At the same time, open its jaw with your right hand.

If there is no one to help you, wrap the cat in a towel with only its head protruding and open its mouth as described above.

The most common cause of choking in cats is bones that lodge sideways in the animal's throat. This can be prevented by not feeding bones to your pet.

Fishhooks

If a cat gets a fishhook caught in its mouth, or anywhere on its body, get the poor creature to a vet at once. It is simple to remove a fishhook after the cat has had a general anesthetic. Unfortunately, most fishhook accidents happen in places remote from vets, so that it may be up to you to remove the hook.

A cat, unlike a dog, does not paw at its throat or mouth if something is caught there. (And that is where puss usually gets the fishhooks caught.) Instead of pawing, cats usually hunch up and keep gulping. Since a cat that has been hurt may run off and hide, the first precaution is to confine the animal. Place a basket or a box with a weight on top of it over the cat while you gather your tools and find an assistant. One assistant will do; two are better; three assistants are ideal.

Preparation: In addition to assistants you will need a

pair of needle-nosed pincers or wire clippers and a sharp knife or razor blade. Boil them for twenty minutes to be certain they are completely sterile. You will also need a thick towel, two short lengths of rope or two neckties, and a bright light to work by.

Procedure: When you have gathered your equipment and are ready to begin the operation, roll the cat tightly in the towel (only its head should protrude), and proceed as follows. One assistant holds the cat in the towel; another assistant knots a necktie around the cat's upper jaw and holds it as steady as possible; the third assistant pries open the cat's lower jaw and knots the other necktie around it, using the necktie to keep the jaw open.

Examine the way the hook is embedded in the cat. Do not try to pull the hook out, or you will tear a bloody chunk out of the animal. Determine which way the barb is pointing, and push it out through the skin. Use the pincers or wire clippers to snip off the head of the hook. Then push it out. (Push in the opposite direction from where the barb is pointing.)

If the hook is embedded in a way that prevents you from getting at its head, use the knife to make an incision over the area where the head of the hook is embedded. Do not be squeamish. Your incision will do much less damage than a forceful pull. After you have made the incision, use the pincers to snip off the head of the hook.

When the hook is out, clean the wound with soap and water, and disinfect it by pouring a solution of hydrogen peroxide directly on the wound. (The hydrogen peroxide will bubble and froth; this is quite natural.) Although the wound is now dressed, do not let the cat go. If it didn't run sooner, after what it's just suffered, it's sure to take off now. It is best to keep the cat confined until it appears to trust you again.

Swallowing Safety Pins or Other Sharp Foreign Objects

Force-feed the cat bread or oatmeal. Also feed it small balls of cotton that have been dipped in meat extract or chicken broth. (See Force-Feeding.) An X ray may be necessary; obtain professional advice.

Tonsillitis—Choking—Foreign Bodies in the Throat

These three conditions produce very similar symptoms.

General symptoms: The cat coughs, licks its lips, appears distressed, and may cry out in pain. It refuses food and may appear apathetic or sleepy. Bones stuck between the larynx and the stomach cause no loss of appetite, but the cat vomits when it eats. There is excessive dribbling and profound depression. There is no home treatment for bones lodged in this area. Consult a veterinarian.

Tonsillitis:

Symptoms: Choking; profound depression; high fever (over 103°F.). (See Taking Temperature.) When you open the cat's mouth, the tonsils (at the back of the throat) will look like two swollen strawberry-colored lumps.

Treatment: Calm the cat with petting and soothing words. Administer one-half of a 250-mg. Tylenol ® tablet, once only. Give no food or water, except for some cracked ice, until a vet has examined the cat. (Put the ice into a perforated bowl—a soap dish with holes punched in it is ideal—so that the cat can moisten its mouth by licking the ice, but cannot drink.) Cats with sore throats have a tendency to vomit anything they swallow. If the cat is allowed to fill its stomach with a quantity of water, it will retch and further irritate its throat. This will make the cat even thirstier, and will set in motion the dangerous drink-vomit cycle.

Foreign body in throat or mouth: Open the cat's mouth and look down its throat with a flashlight. (See How to Open a Cat's Mouth.) If a foreign body (e.g., a bone) is stuck in the throat, use your fingers to pull it out. If it's too far down to reach, use a pair of needlenosed pliers to pull out the object.

3

Problems of the Skin and Hair

SKIN DISEASES

Cats can develop acute skin conditions very quickly. These painful, unhealthy conditions should not be allowed to continue.

The most obvious indication of skin problems is excessive scratching. Any cat that scratches itself constantly either has trouble or is headed in that direction. Prompt treatment by the cat owner can prevent nuisances from becoming serious problems.

Skin diseases also have a public health aspect. Some (e.g., ringworm and sarcoptic mange) can be transmitted from cats to people. Many others are transmitted from animal to animal (e.g., demodectic mange).

For purposes of home treatment, we can divide skin diseases into the following categories: (1) Contagious (transmitted by direct contact). (2) Infectious (can be transmitted through the air (e.g., ringworm). (3) Noninfectious and noncontagious (e.g., eczema and diseases caused by hormonal imbalance).

Contagious: Infestations of mange mites, or ringworm, should be treated under strict hygienic conditions. The affected cat should be kept away from other animals and small children.

Noncontagious: With noncontagious skin diseases, the owner may feel there is not the same urgency for treatment. Some owners, in time, even "learn to live with" their cat's condition. Aside from the eventual worsening of the original complaint, neglect invites a host of secondary complications.

All abnormal skin conditions should be diagnosed and treated at once. In the noncontagious category of skin diseases, perhaps the most common example are warts. These may be due to viruses, but this has not been proved. If you take your pet to a vet when you first observe this growth, it is usually very simple to remove.

Hormonal imbalance: This is a common cause of noncontagious skin disease. The imbalance can produce bald spots as well as certain varieties of eczema in the cat. If the symptoms are observed and treatment instituted early, the condition can be corrected quickly.

Hereditary diseases: Owners of highly bred cats, especially those bred for certain abnormal traits (e.g., the squash-nosed Persian), should be aware of the particular skin diseases their animal is heir to.

External origins: Chemicals, foreign bodies (such as grass seeds), even overexposure to light can cause a skin disease.

Allergies: Probably the most common of noncontagious skin diseases are those caused by allergies. Unfortunately, they are also the most difficult to cure.

Abscesses

An abscess is a swelling caused by a collection of pus under the cat's skin. This swelling, accompanied by localized pain and heat, usually grows larger until "pointing" occurs. Then the abscess softens and, finally, bursts. Cats that fight often get abscesses on their faces, at the root of their tails, or on their feet.

Since an abscess is formed by the body in order to wall off infection, it should not be squeezed. Allow it to burst naturally, thus avoiding breaking down the wall and forcing the infection back into the body.

Treatment: Encourage the abscess to "point" by bathing the abscess in hot saline solution (see Saline Solution), and applying hot compresses directly over the abscess until it bursts. When it does burst, wash the pus away with a solution of 2 teaspoons of hydrogen peroxide added to 1 pint of warm water. To keep an abscess open and draining, bathe it every two hours with a solution of warm salt water (1 teaspoon of table salt to 1 pint of warm water).

The pus that drains from the abscess is usually a creamy color; occasionally, however, it is pink-tinged and large amounts are sometimes confused with hemorrhage.

If the compresses are not effective after twenty-four hours, it may be necessary to lance the abscess. If a vet is not available, the owner may lance the abscess himself.

Technique for lancing: (1) Boil a single-edged razor for twenty minutes. (2) Clean the skin around the affected area with a disinfectant. (3) Have an assistant, wearing heavy gloves, hold the cat's head tightly. (See Restraint and Handling.) (4) Make a half-inch incision over the softest, reddest part of the swelling. (5) Allow the abscess to drain. (6) Dress the wound.

Mange

Mange is a common parasitic skin disease caused by microscopic, spiderlike mites.

Cats are susceptible to four types of mange. In the order of their frequency, they are: otodectic, notoedric, demodectic, and sarcoptic.

Otodectic mange: (See Ear Mites.)

Notoedric mange: This form of mange is highly contagious to other cats although it is easily confused with dermatitis, ringworm, demodectic, and sarcoptic mange. If notoedric mange is suspected, confine the cat and take strict sanitary precautions when treating the animal. A definite diagnosis can be made only after a microscopic examination of skin scrapings.

Symptoms: Constant scratching; breaks in the skin on cat's ears and face; marked loss of hair (bald patches with grayish yellow crusts); skin around infected areas reddens and eventually wrinkles.

Treatment: Apply sulfur and lime washes, or rotenone or sulfur ointments (all available without prescription). Dip a cotton swab or Q-tip ® into the ointment and rub it gently into the infected areas for one minute twice a day. It is also useful to shampoo with a selenium sulfide preparation, once a day for two weeks.

Demodectic mange: This type of mange is quite rare in cats. Its visible symptoms and treatment are the same as those for notoedric mange.

Sarcoptic mange: Symptoms and treatment same as above. This form of mange can affect the cat's entire body, and can be transmitted from cats to people. Strict sanitary precautions should be taken. Throw away any bedding used by the cat. Remove the cat's collar or harness for as long as the condition persists. When you have cured the mange, replace the old collar or harness with a new one. Do not allow the cat to come in contact with other animals; keep your pet indoors. After every treatment, use liberal amounts of soap and water and pHisoDerm ® to thoroughly clean and disinfect the area where you have been treating the cat. Make certain that you dispose of the cotton carefully so that no one will touch it. Wash your hands.

Relief from excessive biting, scratching: Excessive biting and scratching of the infected areas can cause secondary infections and other complications. An Elizabethan collar will prevent scratching. (See Elizabethan Collar.)

Application of soothing, cooling lotion (e.g., calamine lotion) may also provide temporary relief to the irritated areas.

Warning: Never use phenol-based soaps or Lysol ® to wash your cat because cats absorb phenol and Lysol ® through their skins. These preparations will kill the cat's mange and may also kill the cat. Also avoid any soaps or preparations containing coal tar or wood tar derivatives.

Ringworm

Ringworm is a disease of the top layer of the skin (the epidermis) caused by two groups of fungi, both of which are contagious and can affect human beings.

Symptoms: Ringworm is fairly common in cats. Breaks in the skin are accompanied by a collection of gray flakes in the fur that resemble cigarette ash. This stage is followed by characteristic circular, dry, scaly patches.

Treatment: Always wash your hands after treating a cat

suffering from ringworm. Clip the hair around the breaks in the skin. Apply a dilute solution of pHisoDerm ® to the lesions and the surrounding area (1 teaspoon to 10 teaspoons of water). Saturate cotton in the solution, and continue applications for as long as the lesions are visible. Griseofulvin is the treatment of choice (available from vets or doctors).

Although the condition may disappear spontaneously in about two months in healthy cats, do not delay treatment. Ringworm is a highly contagious and very uncomfortable disease and should be treated immediately.

Warts

Small, round, pinkish lumps on the cat's skin, most frequently found around the muzzle at the top of the head.

Cause: Not definitely known. Warts may be caused by a virus, or they may come from kissing frogs. In any case, they are not serious; and since they will not trouble your cat, do not let them trouble you.

Treatment: A wart that has a definite "neck" may be removed: tie it off with a piece of thread. In two to three days, the wart will drop off. Otherwise, warts are easily removed by a veterinarian.

ALLERGIES OF THE SKIN

Allergic Dermatitis

Causes: Food allergies; intestinal parasites; synthetic

carpet fibers; flea saliva; detergents. Causes vary from cat to cat.

Symptoms: Sore, weeping, itchy, red patches along the spine. If left untreated, the condition will not improve.

Treatment: The goal is to break the itch-scratch cycle. Shampoo the cat once a week with a selenium sulfide shampoo (e.g., Seleen ®). Apply liberal amounts of soothing lotions (e.g., calamine lotion) to the affected areas twice a day. To prevent scratching, bandage the cat's feet.

If the allergic dermatitis is caused by fleas, get rid of the fleas as well.

Eczema

A common condition in cats. Eczema is a general term for a superficial inflammation of the skin and occurs in two forms: chronic and acute.

Causes: Improper diet (excess carbohydrate, too little fat); vitamin deficiencies; feeding fish exclusively. (Make certain your cat eats a balanced diet.) Other causes include: allergies; dirty skin; abrasions from collars or harness; friction between the elbow and chest; hormonal imbalance; individual predisposition.

Chronic eczema:

Symptoms: The affected skin becomes dry, flaky, and is darker than the rest of the skin.

Treatment: Identify the cause and correct it wherever possible.

Acute eczema:

Symptoms: Severe itching; broken, sparse hairs around the affected areas; bright red, sore skin. In long-haired breeds the disease may go undetected due to the matting of the animal's coat.

Acute moist eczema:

Symptoms: Acute pain; loss of appetite; depression; constant scratching; sudden appearance of large, wet area exuding serum (a yellow-tinged fluid that dries to a yellow crust). Painful breaks in the skin can appear overnight and are most common in areas that the animal can scratch or lick conveniently. The lesions vary in size from a penny upward; initially, they are wet and purulent, then they dry to a yellow scab.

Treatment: Apply a solution of potassium permanganate crystals to the area—a pinch of crystals (available at drugstores) to a pint of water. Bathe the cat with a shampoo containing selenium sulfide. (See How to Shampoo a Cat.) Dry the animal and dab calamine lotion on the affected areas.

If the irritation persists for more than twenty-four hours, contact a veterinarian.

Labial eczema:

Symptoms: Raw, red lips; brown-stained and foul-smelling hair surrounding the muzzle.

Treatment: Clip the hair around the lips with a pair of round-edged scissors, the type used to clip children's fingernails. You will need an assistant to hold the cat while you do the clipping. (See Restraint and Handling.) Clean the area daily with soap and water. In very severe cases, paint the sore areas with a silver nitrate (caustic) pencil; wear rubber gloves, or you will burn your fingers. If home treatment is not successful, professional attention will be necessary.

Hives (Urticaria)

Rarely seen in cats.

*Causes:*Poison ivy; poison oak; stinging nettles; insect bites or stings; chemicals.

Symptoms: Sudden, acute swelling of cat's eyelids and face; appearance of round, smooth, raised patches on cat's skin; possible fever or vomiting.

Treatment: If the cat is not in great discomfort, treatment may not be necessary. Most cases clear up in six to eight hours. If the condition persists after twenty-four hours, consult a veterinarian.

Miliary Eczema

Causes: This form of eczema results from various hormone deficiencies or feeding the cat too much fish, to the exclusion of other dietary essentials. (See also Eczema)

Symptoms: Severe itching; the owner may notice the cat scratching more than usual; small scabs at the base of the hairs along the spine.

Treatment: Stop feeding the cat fish. If you haven't been feeding fish, suspect a hormone deficiency and get professional help. Bathe the cat with a selenium sulfide shampoo. Even though the cause may be hormonal, the cat will scratch itself and its skin should be kept clean. Shampoo once a week for one month. (See How to Shampoo a Cat.) Administer 50 mg. vitamin C, daily.

If there is no improvement after a week of home treatment, hormone therapy may be required. Seek professional advice.

INJURIES TO THE SKIN

Bee and Wasp Stings

Treatment: If you have seen the insect stinging your cat, try to locate the stinger (it may be at the top of the swelling); remove it by pinching at the bottom of the swelling with a pair of tweezers or a couple of wooden match sticks. Only bee stingers stay in, because they are barbed. Do not try to pull out the stinger with your fingers. You will only succeed in squeezing the balance of its contents into your cat.

Bee stings: Apply baking soda directly to the sting to relieve the pain.

Wasp stings: For wasp stings, use vinegar. For stings on the mouth use an ice pack to reduce the swelling.

Mild cases: Fortunately, most stings are not severe and the pain usually subsides in half an hour. Treat mild discomfort in cats with one-half of a 250-mg. Tylenol ® tablet, within a twenty-four-hour period. If the cat's discomfort lasts longer than a day, professional assistance is necessary.

Severe cases: If the swelling (or swellings) becomes very large (golf-ball size or larger), or if the cat has difficulty in breathing, get the animal to a veterinarian immediately. An injection of an antihistamine is necessary. If a vet isn't available, try an animal-loving doctor, a dentist, even a pharmacist.

Bites, Fighting Wounds

There are two types of wounds received from animal bites: puncture wounds and lacerated wounds.

Puncture wounds: These are small, deep holes in the skin, often accompanied by bruising. Puncture wounds are the most serious kinds of bite wounds and they usually become infected. If a puncture wound is left untreated, the skin will heal but an abscess will form underneath.

Treatment: Clean the area around the wound with soap and water or pHisoDerm ® and water. Consult a veterinarian within twenty-four hours to treat the infection. In severe cases, get professional help immediately.

Lacerated wounds: The wound is jagged; the skin is torn, and there may be profuse bleeding.

Treatment: Clean the wound with hydrogen peroxide or soap and water. Check to be sure that the wound has drained and that no infection remains. If the wound is discharging pus it is still infected. If the wound is very large, it may require stitches. Consult a vet.

Bruises, Contusions

Description: Bruises and contusions are easy to see on the hairless parts of the animal: the bruise is bluish red and painful to the touch. If the bruise is under the fur, you will not be able to see it, but you can feel it and judge by your cat's reaction just how severe it is.

Treatment: Examine the area around the bruise for breaks in the skin; these cuts and abrasions are often seen in association with bruises. If you find any cuts, clean and dress them. (See Wounds.) Apply hot compresses over the bruise for five minutes, every two hours. If possible, have an assistant hold the cat while you are applying the compresses. (See Restraint and Handling.) If the cat is suffering marked discomfort, administer one-half of a 250-mg. Tylenol ® tablet, once only. (See How to Administer Tablets and Pills.)

Burns and Scalds

Burns and scalds are the most common household accidents, and the cat owner should familiarize himself with the treatment of these mishaps *before* they occur.

Causes: A burn is caused by dry heat (e.g., a flame); a scald is caused by moist heat (e.g., steam). The difference is academic, since symptoms and treatment are the same in both conditions.

Treatment: When handling or treating a cat that has been burned, be careful. Burns are very painful and animals in pain resent being handled. An assistant is essential. (See Restraint and Handling.)

In serious cases, treat first for shock by wrapping the cat in a blanket to keep it warm. Then force-feed a solution made by adding 3 teaspoons of dextrose monohydrate to ½ pint of water. (See also Force-Feeding.) Relieve the pain by administering one-half of a 250-mg. Tylenol ® tablet. (See How to Administer Tablets and Pills.) Clean the area around the burn with a dilute solution of hydrogen peroxide (1 teaspoon peroxide to 1 pint of water) to remove any damaged tissue (burned or charred skin). Apply tannic acid jelly (available at drugstores) or a solution of strong, cooled tea to the burned area. Bandage the area to prevent further loss of fluid, which can lead to serious problems. In very severe cases, wrap the animal in a blanket and take it to a vet immediately.

Long-haired cats: Usually takes two to three days before any symptoms appear. Then a sticky green crust forms on the skin. Do not pull this crust off. It will come off naturally, leaving a large, pinkish, weeping area. If it doesn't come away, bathe it or soak it off. Then clean the area, using some cod liver oil on a cotton pad for the dressing.

In very severe cases with associated shock, a vet will administer stimulants and plasma to combat the loss of fluid. (See Shock; Transportation of Injured Cats.)

Cat Falls in a Hot Bath

This happens more frequently than anyone (except a cat owner) would believe. The cause is a combination of the cat's antipathy to water, its overriding curiosity, and the slipperiness of bathtubs. If you draw a hot bath for yourself and if puss can get into the bathroom, then sooner or later . . . splash.

Treatment: If the cat has not jumped out by itself, grab a towel and use it to pull the cat out of the tub. Then, with the cat still wrapped in the towel, plunge it into a sinkful of cold water, or wrap it in another cold, wet towel. The object is to reduce the cat's body temperature as quickly as possible.

If the cat is in a state of shock (semi- or unconscious; pallor of the mucous membranes; shallow breathing), force-feed one-half cup of cooled, strong black coffee. (See Force-Feeding.) Keep the cat wrapped up warmly (after you've cooled its burned tissues), and let it rest.

Any breaks in the skin that appear after the cat's bathtub experience should be treated as moist burns (scalds).

If the cat is in pain, administer one-half of a 250-mg. Tylenol ® tablet. Wait a few hours before giving the cat any food or water.

Chemical Burns

Causes: Caustic soda; sulfuric acid; hydrochloric acid; diesel oil. (Cats often come in contact with diesel oil when they explore under a parked truck.)

Symptoms: A chemical burn resembles a scald. The wound is moist and oozing. The skin around the burn usually sloughs off. If the cat has tried to drink the chemical, there will be sores on its muzzle and tongue.

Treatment: Use mild soap and water to wash the chemical off the cat's fur and skin. For acid burns, apply dilute bicarbonate of soda to the burned area. If the burn was caused by an alkali (e.g., battery acid), apply vinegar to the burned area. If you have no idea which chemical caused the burn, play it safe and clean the burned area with soap and water. Apply hydrogen peroxide directly on the burn to disinfect it.

Fleas

Fleas, like taxes, are a perennial problem for cat owners. Fleas cause your cat intense irritation and discomfort and carry tapeworm eggs. Your cat's fleas may bite you, but you will be glad to know that it is only in passing; these fleas will not live on human beings.

Symptoms: When grooming your cat, if you notice small, reddish, flat creatures running through the fur, your cat has fleas. When the animal's fur is parted, it will look as if tiny particles of black grit have been scattered through the hairs.

Treatment: Bathe the cat with a shampoo containing selenium sulfide (available at drugstores) every three days for two weeks. On the days when the cat is not being bathed, powder the animal thoroughly with a commercial preparation containing rotenone powder (available at drugstores and pet shops).

During the flea season, which varies from place to place, the cat should wear a flea collar (available at pet shops). Change the collar at regular intervals of three to five weeks. Check under collar frequently to be sure cat is not developing a skin irritation. Supplement baths and powderings with commercial aerosol sprays that kill fleas on contact (available at pet shops). Remove collar while bathing or spraying. Although sprays are usually effective, if they don't kill all the fleas, you will have to bathe the cat—a difficult task but not an impossible one. Put the cat into a pillowcase with its head protruding, and wash it through the pillowcase. Dust flea powder around the cat's bed.

Kittens: Kittens under eight weeks of age should not be powdered. Bathe them in a diluted solution of selenium sulfide. Make sure that you wash off all the shampoo after bathing. Dry well.

When defleaing the cat, be sure that the cat's environment, your home, is also free of fleas. To remove fleas from carpets and cushions, spray with any commercial, fly-killing aerosol (available at hardware stores). For heavy infestation, call an exterminator.

Frostbite

In this condition, destruction of tissue is caused by exposure to severe cold. Circulation is affected in the nose, toes, tips of the ears, feet, and tip of the tail.

Mild cases: Frostbitten skin becomes cold and white; loss of hair around the affected areas.

Severe cases: Loss of hair, followed by redness and localized pain.

Most severe cases: Affected area remains sore and sensitive to the touch, swells, then shrivels. Skin around the area sloughs away, leaving an open, weeping surface.

Treatment: In mild cases, increase the circulation of the blood to the frostbitten skin by rubbing the affected area with your hand, then apply camphor oil or oil of wintergreen. If the cat is very uncomfortable, half of a 250-mg. Tylenol ® tablet may be given. (See How to Administer Tablets and Pills.) In extreme cases, amputation may be necessary. (See Gangrene.) Seek professional help for all cases.

Lice

Lice are flat, gray wingless insects sometimes confused with fleas. Fleas run and jump through the cat's fur, but lice crawl slowly through the fur or cling to the base of the hairs.

Although animal lice will not live on human beings,

they carry disease and cause intense irritation to an animal and may lead to serious complications. They should, therefore, be destroyed.

Treatment: Shampoo and bathe the cat twice a week for two weeks with a shampoo containing selenium sulfide (e.g., Seleen ®).

Porcupines

Technique for removing porcupine quills: Use tweezers or a pair of gloves, and remove the quills one at a time: twist each quill one full turn clockwise, then pull—do not jerk—it out.

Skunks

Technique for neutralizing skunk spray: Wash the cat with tomato juice, making sure none gets in the eyes. This will dilute most of the odor.

Skunk spray in eyes: Wash the cat's eyes with clean, cool water. Badly inflamed eyes call for a veterinarian's skill.

Ticks

The tick is a blood-sucking parasite with a shiny, spherical body that varies in size from one-quarter to one-half inch in diameter. It is creamy gray in color, and looks like a soybean with tiny legs at one end.

Country animals often come into contact with the

common sheep or wood tick. Usually, ticks are first seen when you are grooming your cat—another good reason for frequent grooming.

Treatment: Do not try to pull the tick out. Ticks have powerful sucking jaws that burrow into the cat's skin. If you try to pull the tick out, its head may break off, leaving its mouth under the cat's skin, and a sinus (a small puncture wound that does not heal) may eventually develop. The trick is to get the tick to remove its mouth before you pull it off your cat. There are three techniques for accomplishing this: (1) Pour a little ether or lighter fluid on a pad of cotton, and place the pad over the tick for half a minute. Pull the tick out. (2) Coat each tick with Vaseline ®, then remove it with tweezers. (3) Hold the lighted end of a cigarette very close to the tick, without actually touching it or the cat. The heat will make the tick withdraw its head and it may then be removed.

If the head of the tick breaks off, clean the skin around the area with pHisoDerm ® or soap and water. Use a boiled (sterile) needle to remove the head of the tick from under the cat's skin, exactly as you would remove a splinter from your own finger. Dress the wound with a poultice.

In tick-infested areas, keep the cat free of ticks by bathing once a month in a .0012 solution of gamma bene-zene hexachloride (available from drugstores). Be sure to wash all of the solution off the animal's fur after bathing, since this solution can be poisonous to cats. (See Restraint and Handling.) Buy a flea and tick collar for the cat.

Wounds

A wound is a break (lesion) in the body surfaces. When the wound occurs, the cat bleeds. Usually, if the wound is superficial and the bleeding slight, clotting will occur and the bleeding will stop. But if the cat is losing a lot of blood, first aid must be administered.

Treatment: The first priority is to stop the bleeding, regardless of whether or not it is arterial or venous. If the animal is bleeding very badly, don't waste time; jam a wad of rags, Kleenex ®, or a towel over the wound, press hard, and hold the wad of material there until the bleeding stops. If nothing else is available, use your hand or fingers pressed directly on the wound to stop the bleeding.

Once you have stanched the wound, try to determine whether the bleeding is arterial or venous. If the blood is bright red and spurting, it comes from a severed artery. If the blood is a deeper red and oozing, it comes from a vein. For arterial wounds, apply a tourniquet between the wound and the heart. For venous wounds, the tourniquet is applied on the side of the wound farthest from the heart.

If the wound is on the trunk or the neck, where a tourniquet cannot be used, keep pressing the wad of material (or your hand) over the wound until the bleeding stops. When you do remove the pressure, be careful not to tear away the protective clotting and start the bleeding again.

Once the bleeding has been controlled, the next step depends upon the severity of the injury and whether the cat is in a state of shock.

Dressing the wound: Clip the hair around the wound with blunt-pointed scissors. Wash the wound with mild soap and cooled, boiled water. If you have an antiseptic handy (e.g., pHisoDerm ® or hydrogen peroxide), apply it. Be sure to wash away any dirt, oil, or grease from the center of the wound. After drying, apply a simple dressing to keep out infection: a pad of cotton properly secured with adhesive tape will do. Change the dressing once a day. For severe wounds, after cleaning and dressing, contact your veterinarian.

The most efficacious treatment for a wound can be determined by observing the kind of wound it is.

Classification of wounds: (1) Clean, *incised wounds* bleed freely; a pressure bandage or tourniquet may be applied. (2) *Lacerated wounds* are jagged, irregular wounds that bleed minimally and require ordinary bandaging. (3) *Puncture wounds* are usually caused by bites and are nearly always infected. (See Abscesses.) (4) *Contused wounds* include any of the above types of wounds accompanied by surrounding bruises. In addition to washing and disinfecting the wound, hot compresses should be applied. (See Bruises, Contusions; Compresses—Hot and Cold.)

THE HAIR

Baldness (Alopecia)

Causes: This condition is not uncommon in cats and may occur without any visible cause. It may be inherited or acquired. Acquired baldness may be the result of an iodine deficiency, a hormonal imbalance, dietary deficiencies, general infectious diseases, chemical poisoning, gastroenteritis, or pneumonia.

Symptoms: Hair falls out in patches, which may or may not itch.

Treatment: Apply a solution of 1 teaspoon of iodine

crystals to 1 pint of glycerin. Shake well until the crystals have dissolved. Saturate a bit of cotton with the solution and apply directly to the bald patches. Continue treatment for five to six weeks. If there is no improvement, obtain professional help for diagnosis and treatment.

Dandruff (Scurf)

This condition is common in cats with dry coats. Cat's dandruff looks exactly like human dandruff: fine, white flakes scattered throughout the coat, especially along the spine.

Treatment: This skin condition should be promptly treated to prevent it from becoming a problem. Shampoo the cat once a week for four weeks with a selenium sulfide shampoo (e.g., Seleen ®).

The amount of difficulty experienced in shampooing a cat depends primarily upon the cat: some cats will co-operate, others will not. An animal that is accustomed to being handled and groomed is more likely to permit a shampoo without too much fuss.

Unruly cats require an assistant who can scruff the cat (See Restraint and Handling) while you do the shampooing. Be careful not to get soap in the animal's eyes, or it will be twice as difficult next time. If there is no one to help you, put the cat into a pillowcase (only its head protruding) and shampoo it through the pillowcase. Feed the cat 1 teaspoon of corn oil daily for one week.

Cats with a tendency toward dandruff should have regular amounts of corn oil added to their diets: 1 table-spoon of corn oil a week should prevent the condition from recurring.

Paint Removal

Technique: Get some dry cloths and rub off all the paint you can. Wash small areas thoroughly with soap and water and keep rubbing with dry cloths. Snip off patches of matted hair with scissors. For particularly difficult patches, pour a little rubbing alcohol on the patch; rub off with a dry cloth.

Warning: Never use kerosene, turpentine, or any of the paint solvents; they may cause burns on the cat's skin.

Lead in paints: Paints that contain lead are poisonous when ingested. If a cat has eaten paint with a lead base, or has licked lead paint off its coat, force-feed a bowl of milk with two egg whites beaten into it. (See Force-Feeding.) If lead poisoning is suspected, do not try to induce vomiting. If the cat is in pain, or is covered with paint, get it to a veterinarian immediately.

A cat with paint on its fur will try to lick the paint off. Although it probably won't succeed in getting all the paint off, it probably will succeed in licking off enough to poison itself. (See also Poisoning.)

Often, a cat covered with paint may require a general anesthetic so that the fur can be combed out or clipped. In severe cases, the pain caused by paint on the skin can drive the cat into a state of shock, requiring intravenous fluids and other professional treatment.

Shedding (Loss of Hair)

A certain degree of shedding is natural, occurring twice a year, during the spring and autumn. However, this shedding schedule is often altered in cats living mostly indoors during the winter. If the cat loses large amounts of hair at other times, make sure that the animal is being properly groomed. If regular grooming has been carried out, this excessive loss of hair should be considered abnormal.

Causes: Excess shedding may be due to a thyroid deficiency; chronic nephritis; malnutrition; hormone deficiency; fatty acid deficiency; or fear.

Treatment: If the shedding is not due to a specific disease, bathe and groom the cat, using a shampoo containing selenium sulfide (e.g., Seleen ®). (See How to Shampoo a Cat.) Add one teaspoon of corn oil a week to the shedding cat's diet.

4

Problems of
the Chest

ALLERGIES OF THE RESPIRATORY TRACT

Asthma

This is not a common condition but, when it does occur, it must be treated; it can develop into something more serious.

Symptoms: Affected cats become short-winded and wheezy. Usually occurs during the summer months.

Treatment: Can be controlled with medication. Consult a veterinarian.

Hay Fever

Hay fever, an allergy of the upper respiratory tract, nose and throat, is fairly common in cats.

104

Symptoms: Sneezing, running eyes and nose, during periods of high pollen count. (Dates vary with the locale.)

Treatment: Professional treatment is required.

BRONCHITIS, EXCESSIVE COUGHING

Bronchitis is an acute or chronic inflammation of the bronchial tubes.

Symptoms: Coughing spasms, often with mucus; sometimes accompanied by a high fever.

Treatment: Examine the cat's throat under a bright light, to make sure that the cough is not caused by a foreign object in the mouth or throat. (See How to Open a Cat's Mouth.) Treat the symptoms as they arise. For the cough, give a mixture of 1 teaspoon of glycerin mixed with 1 teaspoon of honey three times a day. You will probably have to pour this down the cat's throat. (See Force-Feeding.)

Diet: No food for twenty-four hours; then, a light diet of fish or chicken. If your cat is still coughing excessively after forty-eight hours, consult a veterinarian.

If there is no fever, administer diphenhydramine hydrochloride elixir (e.g., Benadryl ®, Hydrillin ®), 1 teaspoon twice a day for three days.

If you think your cat has bronchitis, contact a vet. Home treatment should be attempted only in extraordinary circumstances, when professional help is not available.

CHEST WOUNDS

Treatment: Place a moistened gauze pad or wad of material directly over the wound. Place a plastic bag or sheet of plastic over the pad and secure it with adhesive or Scotch ® tape, to obtain an airtight shield over the wound.

In an emergency, do not waste time looking for a pad or wad of material. Put your hand or fingers directly on the bleeding wound and press. This should stop the bleeding until you can dress the wound properly.

If the wound continues to bleed through the dressing, do not remove the dressing; this will disturb the blood clot that is forming over the wound and increase the bleeding. Apply another pad and bandage it tighter, or apply more pressure by hand over the wound.

Transporting a cat with a chest wound: Move a wounded cat only if absolutely necessary. If you can hear the air sucking in and out of a wound, carry the cat on its breastbone. Otherwise, carry the animal with the wound uppermost.

COLDS

Cats do not catch colds. But if a cat exhibits the symptoms of the common cold, do not treat these signs lightly. The symptoms (running eyes and nose, coughing, shivering, etc.) suggest a more serious ailment. (See Flu; Sinusitis; Pneumonia.) Seek professional advice.

Flu (Feline Viral Rhinotracheitis—FVR)

All cats are susceptible to cat flu, but the exotic breeds (e.g., Siamese, Burmese, Abyssinian, Rex) are particularly sensitive and, in very severe cases, may die. At present, there is no effective vaccine available. Although it is a highly contagious disease, cat flu cannot be transmitted to human beings or to other animal species, only to other cats.

Symptoms: The incubation period is from two to four days. The onset of the infection is marked by slight fever, sneezing, excessive salivation (drooling), and lethargy. Initially, the cat's temperature may reach 105°F., then fluctuate between normal and 103°F. for the course of the disease: up to three weeks. The next stage is marked by a clear discharge from the eyes and nose. After a day or so the discharge becomes yellow, sticky and particularly noticeable on the chest and paws, where the animal has tried to rub the stickiness away. The cat also loses its appetite and becomes depressed.

During the course of cat flu, there is progressive dehydration and raw sores appear on the tongue and in the mouth. Even after a satisfactory recovery, the cat may be left with a chronic sinus infection, which produces a chronic, yellowish mucous discharge from the nose.

Treatment: Since cat flu is a viral infection, and viruses do not respond to antibiotics, there is no simple cure for the disease. The cat's owner can only treat the symptoms as they arise.

Although a veterinarian must be consulted, proper supportive home treatment is important. Bathe the cat's eyes and nose with warm water to remove the accumulating discharge. To prevent dehydration and starvation, administer (force-feed if necessary) 5 tablespoons dextrose monohydrate to 1 pint of water (up to ¼ pint a day) and a meat extract (up to ¼ pint a day). (See also Force-Feeding.)

Pleurisy

Pleurisy is an inflammation of the membrane (pleura) that surrounds the lungs and lines the walls of the chest.

Symptoms: Same symptoms as pneumonia (i.e., high fever; painful, difficult breathing; loss of appetite; lethargy).

Treatment: Pleurisy, like pneumonia, cannot be accurately diagnosed or adequately treated by the nonprofessional. Home treatment consists of keeping the cat warm and trying to get it to take some nourishment and to drink plenty of fluids. Pleurisy is a serious illness. Therefore, even a suspicion of pleurisy warrants an immediate consultation with a vet.

Pneumonia

Pneumonia is an inflammation of the lungs that is quite common in cats.

Causes: Viruses, bacteria, or worms. A simple chill or cold, if left untreated, may develop into pneumonia.

Symptoms: Coughing; lethargy and dullness; high fever; rattling and bubbling in the chest. Check the cat for bluish-tinged mucous membranes. Often, the afflicted cat will lie on its breastbone, its elbows stuck out at a 45° angle. This is caused by the sore chest that accompanies the disease. When the cat is picked up, there is further evidence of pain in its chest: lifting the animal compresses the lungs and increases their soreness.

Treatment: Pneumonia is a serious disease and immediate professional assistance is necessary. If a veterinarian is not immediately available, the cat owner must make certain that the animal is kept warm. Wrap it in a blanket or a woolen sweater, or button a cardigan around it. Make sure that the room where the cat is kept is warm; also check to see that there is adequate fresh air. Try to tempt the cat's appetite with light, nourishing foods. Give plenty of fluids.

5

Problems of the Abdomen

THE STOMACH

Flatulence (Breaking Wind)

Causes: Overweight; underexercise; dietary imbalance; bowel infection.

Treatment: If your older cat is eating one large meal a day, start feeding it two or three smaller meals daily. Do not overfeed. Remove liver, heart, and milk from the animal's diet. Allow the cat more opportunity for exercise. If the cat is always indoors, get toys (mechanical mice, marbles, etc.) and play with your pet.

If reducing the size of the meals and increasing the chances for more exercise do not remedy the condition, add a teaspoon of charcoal to the cat's food each day.

Occasionally, a cat will break wind excessively and will suddenly become quite bloated. Its abdomen is hard and swollen with gas. This is an emergency: death from *torsion* (twisted stomach) may result. Do not poke or probe the distended abdomen. Get the cat to a veterinarian immediately.

Hair Balls

Cause: Hair balls usually occur in long-haired cats that are not being properly groomed. When the cat licks itself, it swallows the loose hairs that have not been brushed and combed out of its coat. In most cases, these hairs are regurgitated; if this does not happen, the hair accumulates in the cat's stomach.

Symptoms: Sporadic vomiting; straining to pass feces; occasional constipation.

Treatment: In most cases, the cat will eventually pass the hair balls. In acute cases, where there is continual vomiting after eating, administer carefully 2 tablespoons of mineral oil once a week. (See Force-Feeding.)

Prevention: The best method of prevention is the most obvious one—brush and comb your pet regularly. (See Grooming.) Continue to administer 1 tablespoon of mineral oil once a week to long-haired breeds.

Hiccups

Causes: Common in kittens that bolt their food. They also get hiccups when their stomachs are empty. Occasionally, the adult cat will develop hiccups.

Kittens: There is no need to worry about hiccups in

kittens. If the kitten appears distressed, put a little olive oil on your finger and gently rub the kitten's abdomen to induce burping. The olive oil lubricates the fur, reduces friction and possible irritation, and encourages deeper penetration.

Adult cats: The condition is not serious and usually disappears naturally. If the hiccups persist for more than half an hour, administer 1 tablespoon of milk of magnesia. (See Force-Feeding.)

ABDOMINAL DISORDERS

Swelling of the Abdomen

A sudden and dramatic increase in the size of the abdomen suggests: overeating; pregnancy; tumors; fluid in the abdomen; pyometra; ovarian cyst; enlargement of the liver; enlargement of the spleen.

If the symptoms described under these entries (see Index) are similar to those exhibited by your cat, consult a veterinarian. Although the first signs of these conditions may not constitute an emergency, your alertness can help to prevent the serious complications that may develop.

Gastroenteritis

Gastroenteritis is a general term for an infection of the stomach and the intestines.

Symptoms: Vomiting and diarrhea.

Fever stage: High fever; pain; loss of appetite; lethargy; depression.

A cat with a high fever will have dull eyes, a dry, hot nose and a dry coat. Cats with abdominal pain often lie with their hind legs up and their forelegs extended. They seem restless and tend to seek out cold places (e.g., cement floors) to lie on.

Vomiting stage: Continual vomiting. Initially, the vomit is white and frothy; later it is yellow; in an advanced stage, it may be bloodstained. During the vomiting stage the cat will be very thirsty. It will drink and then vomit, setting in motion the drink-vomit cycle.

Diarrhea stage: Once the vomiting stage has been established, diarrhea usually begins. About twenty-four hours later, it becomes bloodstained.

Treatment: Withhold food and water for twenty-four hours. No milk should be given for one week. (See also Diarrhea; Vomiting.)

Hernia

A hernia is the protrusion of internal tissue through a natural opening (e.g., the navel), which would normally close in the course of growth. There are four types of hernia: umbilical, inguinal, scrotal, traumatic.

Umbilical hernia:

Symptoms: Seen fairly frequently in kittens. There is a small protrusion (about one-quarter of an inch) of the intestinal fat visible at the navel.

Treatment: This form of hernia is not usually serious if the amount of tissue protruding is small (one-quarter inch or less). If the protrusion remains small as the kitten grows, leave it alone. If the protruding portion is long, the kitten should be taken to the veterinarian for minor surgery.

Inguinal hernia:

Symptoms: More common in females; most queens have tiny inguinal hernias that never require surgery. Treatment is required when there is a swelling in the groin, which may continue to grow if left untreated.

Treatment: Surgical.

Scrotal hernia:

Symptoms: Occurs only in tomcats. In this form there is a swelling on the right side of the scrotum that is particularly noticeable after the cat has eaten a heavy meal. There may be discomfort and, in severe cases, acute pain and possible strangulation of the bowel. This occurs when the bowel pushes its way through the herniated hole and becomes compressed, twisted, or squashed.

The seriousness of the condition may be assessed by the severity of the pain. In addition to obvious discomfort, there will be pain in the area of the groin. When diagnosing scrotal hernia, be careful not to confuse it with an abscess. Although there is swelling in both conditions, an abscess will be hot and painful to the touch.

Treatment: Surgical.

Emergency: If the pain is acute, seek professional assistance immediately. The danger lies in the possible strangulation of the bowel, which can cause gangrene of the large intestine.

Traumatic hernia (rupture):

Symptoms: Occurs after accidents and appears as a fluctuating swelling, usually on the abdomen.

Treatment: Surgical.

Internal Hemorrhage

Causes: Highway accidents; falls; ingesting anticoagulant poisons (e.g., warfarin, a mouse and rat poison).

Symptoms: Same as those in cases of severe shock (pronounced weakness and heavy panting; fast (140+), weak pulse rate (see Taking the Pulse); pale mucous membranes around the lips and nose; cold paws).

Treatment: There is no home treatment for this condition, since the only certain way of controlling the bleeding is surgically. Wrap the cat in a blanket and get it to a veterinarian. If possible, have someone telephone the vet first, so that he can make the necessary preparations for your arrival.

Intestinal Protrusion

Cats involved in fights or a variety of accidents (e.g., car accidents, jumping onto fences) may tear the abdominal wall and cause the internal organs to protrude. This is a serious emergency, but need not be fatal. The real danger lies in the possibility of shock or accidental self-mutilation. Immediate first aid can prevent these complications.

Treatment: Assess the damage: if a veterinarian is not available, be prepared to do more than just bandage the wound. Calm the cat: try not to touch the wound more than necessary. If the protruding portions of the intestines are dirty, they should be washed gently in boiled water that has been cooled. Pour the water over the protruding part of the intestines. If only a small portion protrudes, gently push it back into the cat's abdomen through the wound. Place a sterile gauze pad over the wound and bandage it around the cat's body. Treat the animal for shock if necessary. (See Shock.) Seek professional help immediately.

6

Problems of the Anorectal Region

ABNORMAL STOOLS

An abnormal bowel movement is distinguished from a normal one by: (1) *Texture:* Hard (constipation); soft (diarrhea). (2) *Color:* Blood in feces; too pale; too dark. (3) *Quantity:* More than usual; less than usual. (4) *Unusual objects in feces:* Worms, bits of bone, etc. (5) *Odor:* Particularly foul.

The signs of abnormal bowel movements are rarely seen alone; they usually appear in conjunction with other symptoms. The cat owner should be aware of the signs listed above. Any one of these symptoms may signal a serious condition and the cat owner should be prepared to seek professional advice quickly.

Blood in Stools

A small amount of blood in the feces is seen from time to time in all meat-eating animals. Larger amounts of blood are not normal and should not be ignored.

Causes: Blood in the feces may be the result of anal impaction (e.g., bones), or may be caused by rectal tumors or accidents. Consider the source or location of the bleeding when attempting to "diagnose" the cause.

Symptoms: Bright red, fresh blood coming from the anal region; black blood coming from the intestines.

Treatment: Unless the cause can be easily identified and treated (e.g., a simple cut), have the veterinarian examine the cat. Give no food until bleeding stops.

Constipation

Causes: Occurs in cats that are fed chicken or fish bones, and in cats with abdominal or rectal tumors, slipped disks, and pelvic fractures.

Symptoms: Straining; passing watery brown stools; bleeding from the anus; vomiting.

Treatment: Administer 1 tablespoon of mineral oil (an excellent laxative) and stop feeding the cat bones. (See Force-Feeding.) The cause of the constipation may be more serious and an enema may be necessary. (See Enema.) If the cat does not have a bowel movement within twenty-four hours, contact a veterinarian. If constipation is suspected in cats which usually go out-of-doors, it will be necessary to confine the cat to the house so that its litter tray may be inspected.

Diarrhea

This is the name given to an abnormal bowel condition in which loose, unformed feces are passed.

Causes: Since cats are natural scavengers, they often suffer mild attacks of diarrhea as a result of eating decayed food. Diarrhea can also be the result of faulty diet, bacteria, viruses, intestinal parasites, or poison.

Symptoms: Frequent passage of loose bowel movements; foul-smelling feces; sometimes associated with vomiting.

Treatment: All food and water should be withheld for twenty-four hours. After twenty-four hours, feed a cup of water a day and small amounts of chicken (deboned) or fish and rice for the next two to three days. Be sure that the chicken or fish is well mixed with the rice, so that the cat will have to eat the rice in order to get the food it likes. *No milk should be given for one week.*

If the diarrhea persists, starve the cat for another twenty-four hours. Then feed the following mixture: 3-4 tablespoons of dextrose monohydrate, 1 raw egg white, a pinch of salt and ½ pint of warm water. Feed the cat 2 tablespoons of this mixture every two hours for two days. (See Force-Feeding.) Put the animal on a diet of deboned chicken or fish and rice for the next two to three days before resuming normal feeding.

Persistent diarrhea: If the diarrhea persists for more than forty-eight hours, it may be the symptom of a more serious disease. Consult a veterinarian without delay.

Sore anus: Cats with diarrhea may develop a sore anus. Apply Vaseline ® or cold cream to soothe the irritated area.

Prolapse of the Rectum

This condition is fairly common in kittens suffering from persistent diarrhea; occasionally it is also seen in older cats.

Treatment: Wash your hands, then gently bathe the area around the anus with warm, soapy water. Apply mineral oil liberally around the anal area. Gently push the protruding portion back until the anus is normal. Contact the vet.

WORMS (See also *Problems of the Skin and Hair*)

Worms are one of several types of parasites that may try to use your cat as their host. Unpleasant as they are, they rarely cause serious problems, except in kittens. During the first eight months of a kitten's life, its owner should be alert to the possibility of worms: the parasites can deplete the kitten's strength and lower its resistance to disease.

Causes: Transmitted by other animals; from feces of affected animals.

Kittens: The following symptoms may be seen separately or in combination: coughing; vomiting of worms; worms in the feces; potbelly; halitosis; stunted growth.

Adult cats: Worms are rarely detected until they are either coughed up or appear in the feces.

Warning: Although most types of worms are not particularly dangerous to the cat itself, the roundworm can be transmitted to humans and may cause blindness. This is one good reason children should not be encouraged to let stray kittens lick their faces. They should be instructed to wash their hands after playing with any animals, including their own.

Since the cat owner cannot make a correct diagnosis of hookworm, whipworm, roundworm, etc., it is advisable to treat all worms and suspected worm conditions with hygienic precaution.

Treatment: For worms other than tapeworms, administer piperazine tablets (available from pet shops or vets), 500 mg. per 10 pounds body weight. Repeat after one week. (See How to Administer Tablets and Pills.)

Tapeworms

When freshly passed, tapeworm segments are flat, narrow, whitish, about one-quarter inch long, moist, and quite active. They dry rapidly and shrivel up. When dry, they resemble small, brownish grains of rice, and are often found in the cat's bedding.

Symptoms: Tapeworms rarely cause any severe symptoms, apart from: a change in the texture and color of the cat's coat; colic; reduced appetite; nervousness; mild diarrhea. The observant owner will notice segments of tapeworms in the feces, and other segments stuck to the fur around the anus.

Treatment: Fortunately, treatment is simple and usually effective. There are a number of excellent medications available that contain dichlorophen (e.g., Dicestol ®, or Teniathane ®). Administer 500 mg. per 6 pounds of body weight after a meal. Wait seven days, then repeat the dose. Since tapeworm eggs are carried by fleas, get rid of the fleas as well as the tapeworms. (See Fleas.)

7

Problems of the Urinary System

Bladder Infection (Cystitis)

A fairly common condition in the cat.

Symptoms: The classic symptom of cystitis in the cat is seen when the animal is in its litter box straining to pass urine. The position is exactly the same as when trying to have a bowel movement, but the constipated cat rarely strains. Other symptoms include: blood or traces of blood in the urine; passing small amounts of urine; abdominal pain. In later stages, the urine is heavily bloodstained. As the disease worsens, pure blood will be passed.

Unfortunately for home diagnosis, cats are so discreet in their urination habits that traces of blood passed in their urine may escape the owner's notice.

Treatment: If cystitis is suspected, do not feed the cat until professional help is available. If it takes longer than twenty-four hours to get to a vet, allow the cat access to all the water it can drink. Keep its drinking bowl full. (See Urethral Obstructions and Bladder Stones.)

There is evidence that the feeding of dry cat foods may be responsible for severe cystitis. Magnesium salts in these commercial preparations may cause sedimentation in the urine and possible subsequent urethral obstruction.

Chronic Interstitial Nephritis (Kidney Failure)

This condition is frequently seen in elderly cats (seven years or older).

Symptoms: Halitosis; constant thirst; pale, watery urine in larger quantities than usual; dull coat; skin eruptions. As the condition progresses, the animal vomits frequently and suffers from diarrhea.

The disease occurs in two forms: compensated and decompensated. In the compensated form, the cat drinks excessively and is able to flush the poison through the kidneys. In the decompensated form, the cat is unable to flush the accumulated poisons out of its body and may die (toxemia and uremia).

Treatment: The cat must be given as much clean water as it can drink. Make sure that its water bowl is always full. Feed the cat a low-protein diet consisting of the white meat from deboned chicken, or fish, or a commercially prepared nephritis diet, available from veterinarians. Antibiotic treatment may also be helpful, but must be left to the discretion of the veterinarian.

Urethral Obstructions and Bladder Stones (Cystic Calculi)

The urethra is the tube running from the bladder through which urine is passed. Occasionally, this tube becomes irritated or, in severe cases, blocked. This condition is more prevalent in tomcats. Blockage of the urethra is serious and must be treated immediately.

Causes: Depending upon the seriousness of the symptoms, this condition could be caused by mild cystitis infection, bladder stones, or complete blockage of the urethra.

Symptoms: Inability to pass urine; squatting in the litter box, as though constipated; distended abdomen; profound depression.

Treatment: There is no home treatment for this condition. You must get professional help immediately. Do not attempt to prod the distended abdomen: the bladder may rupture. If this happens, the cat will die.

8

Problems of
the Extremities

Amputation

Amputation is the removal of one or more limbs either surgically or traumatically.

Surgical amputation: Severe fractures, bone cancer, or very severe cases of arthritis sometimes make amputation necessary. Many cat owners are understandably reluctant to allow this operation, even when the cat's life is at stake. Some would apparently rather have their pets "put away" than have them hobbling about on three legs. If this reluctance is analyzed, it usually turns out that the main objection is to "the way it will look." Cat owners faced with this decision should be made to know that cats learn quite rapidly to compensate for the missing limb and are able to manage very well on three legs. As for appearances, it's amazing how quickly even the most "sensitive" cat owner becomes accustomed to kitty's lack of an appendage.

Traumatic amputation: This occurs after accidents. A

tourniquet must be applied immediately. Then wrap the cat in a towel or coat to keep it warm and minimize the effects of shock while the cat is being transported to the vet. (See Transportation of Injured Cats; Tourniquets.) Put the cat in a box or basket; if driving alone, place the box on the floor of the car. If possible, have someone telephone the vet, so that he can have the necessary transfusions ready when the cat arrives.

Cracked Pads

Symptoms: Cats suffering from cracked pads will be lame on sidewalks and other hard surfaces, but will walk on grass without limping.

Treatment: Examine the paw carefully under a bright light. Make sure that the trouble is not caused by a cut pad. Also check to be sure that the cat's lameness is not the result of a cracked claw. Treat the simple cracked or sore pad by bathing it in a solution of strong, cooled tea (tannic acid) and 4 tablespoons of witch hazel. Pour the mixture into a bowl, put the cat's foot into the bowl and let it soak for a few minutes (or as long as the cat will allow). Do this twice a day for three days. Rub olive oil, baby oil, or lanolin into the cracked pad three times a day for three days. In general, if cut or cracked pads are not bleeding, the less treatment the better.

Dislocations

Dislocations occur when a bone has become displaced (pulled away) from the joint. They should not be confused with fractures, which are broken bones. Unlike fractures, most dislocations should not be splinted.

Symptoms: While a fractured limb tends to swing freely, a dislocated limb is more rigid. There is usually pain and swelling around the dislocated joint and the leg may point in an odd direction, especially in the case of a dislocated elbow. If the cat attempts to walk on the dislocated leg, the leg may support some of the weight before giving way.

Treatment: Do not bandage dislocated limbs. Take the animal to a veterinarian.

Dislocated hip joint: If the dislocated hip cannot be corrected in four to six weeks, a false joint formed of scar tissue will develop; this will work as well as the original. A dislocation must not, however, be left to nature; consult a vet immediately.

Foreign Bodies in the Foot: Punctures

Foreign bodies in the foot pads are usually pieces of glass that cut the pad and work their way into the paw, or pieces of grit that have found their way into existing breaks.

Symptoms: Acute lameness; hobbling; chewing at foot. In later stages, the affected foot will be hot and swollen and the skin of the pad will be shiny. There may be pus coming from the puncture caused by the foreign object.

Treatment: Examine the cat's foot carefully under a bright light. Have an assistant wrap the cat in a towel, with its head and affected paw protruding. Sterilize a needle by boiling it for twenty minutes, then carefully probe the hole until the foreign object is visible. With the aid of tweezers, remove the object. Use the same technique as you would for removing a splinter from your own foot. There is no need to bandage the wound. Pour a solution of hydrogen peroxide directly on the wound.

If probing with the needle does not remove the foreign body, prepare a kaolin poultice (see Poultices) and apply to the affected pad for two days. Keep the poultice in place by bandaging it to the cat's leg; change the poultice and bandage twice a day for two days. (See Bandaging the Leg.) This should draw the object out, or at least make it easier for you to remove it with your needle and tweezers.

Lameness

In cases of severe lameness, the cat owner should seek professional help if it is available. Improperly diagnosed fractures and dislocations can lead to severe complications. (See Limping.)

Causes: Some general rules in diagnosing causes of sudden lameness follow: (1) If the cat is severely lame and the limb is free-swinging, then the leg is probably fractured. (2) If there is displacement (i.e., if the leg is not in its usual position), the leg may be dislocated. (3) If the affected limb is neither free-swinging nor displaced, a strain, sprain or bite should be suspected, or there may be a foreign body or a cut in the pad.

More gradual and more permanent forms of lameness that are caused by arthritis or neoplasms (cancerous growths) may be encountered in the elderly cat.

Treatment: If the lameness persists for more than a few days, consult a veterinarian. It may be possible to cure the condition by surgical treatment or, if the condition is inoperable, the vet may prescribe painkillers.

Limping

Causes: There are several possible causes for limping in cats. If the cause is in the foot, the cat may lick the offending paw. (See Lameness.)

Get the cat into a bright light and carefully examine the paw for thorns, tacks, or small cuts. It is easier to do this when the paw is wet: the hairs lie flat and the thorn or cut is more readily seen. If it isn't a thorn or a cut that is causing the limp, look for a cracked pad. You may not be able to see the cracks, so gently palpate the pad with your thumb. A cracked pad is very sensitive and pressure is painful; be prepared for the cat's reaction. It is helpful to have an assistant hold the cat while you make the examination. If you are alone, wrap the cat in a towel with head and affected paw protruding. Check for a broken claw or a foreign body (splinter, glass, grit) in the pads.

The limp may also be the result of a sprain or a bite. If it is a sprain, there will be pain and heat in the area of the paw. Swelling occurs two to three hours after the sprain or bite. If the limp is the result of a bite, a puncture wound may be visible at the site.

In an older cat, if there is no evidence of a sprain or an injury of the paw, the limp may be caused by arthritis. To decide whether it is arthritis, observe the cat for a few days, and attempt to find the answers to the following questions: (1) Does the cat have difficulty in rising in the morning? Does it move more easily later in the day? (2) Does a change in the weather bring a variation in the lameness? (3) Is the cat unable to jump up or to climb stairs? (4) Is it lame at a walk? At a gallop? (5) Does the lameness grow worse with exercise? (6) Is the lameness intermittent?

Treatment: An arthritic condition is not an emergency. Eventually, however, a cat that continually limps must be seen by a veterinarian. The answers to the above questions will assist the vet in making a correct diagnosis.

As a broad rule of thumb, if the answer to questions (1), (2), and (3) is yes, the cat is probably suffering from arthritis. If the answer to questions (4), (5), and (6) is yes, the cause of the limping is probably traumatic (i.e., the limp has been caused by an accident such as a sprain, a cut, or a bite).

Rickets

Symptoms: Rickets affects kittens from three weeks to six months of age. The first sign is usually a noticeable swelling of the wrist joint. Swellings will also be observed along the side of the chest. Severe cases will eventually develop bending of the long leg bones, causing bow-leggedness.

Causes: Rickets is the result of calcium, phosphorus, and vitamin D deficiencies.

Treatment: Administer one 25-mg. calcium gluconate tablet (available at drugstores) twice a day for one month. Mix sterilized bone flour (available at pet stores and from the vet) into the cat's food. Use multivitamin drops in the strength used for human babies: 2 to 3 drops daily in the cat's food. Seek professional help.

Administration of cod-liver oil is not recommended for young cats suffering from rickets, since cod-liver oil can remove the calcium from the bones if given in excess of 2 to 3 drops daily.

Sprains and Strains

Sprains and strains are very similar in their effect and symptoms. A *sprain* involves the ligaments around a joint; a *strain* involves the muscles. In both cases, the tissues are torn.

Causes: Sprains and strains are usually caused by violent exercise.

Symptoms: The diagnosis must often be made as the result of negative findings for fractures, dislocations, and bites. After these have been eliminated as the cause of the cat's lameness, look for a slight swelling around the joint or muscle.

Treatment: Alternate hot and cold compresses over the swelling until it subsides. If the cat is very uncomfortable, administer analgesics. (See Analgesics.)

Tar on the Feet

An occasional nuisance for owners of adventurous cats.

Treatment: Bathe the cat's feet with a mixture of equal quantities of warm saltwater and olive oil. Soak a wad of cotton in the mixture and gently rub the tar off the cat's feet. (See Restraint and Handling, if necessary.) Whatever tar does not wash off during the foot bath should come off when you dry the cat's feet with a rag. If all the tar doesn't come off after the first washing and drying, repeat the process.

9

Problems of
the Back

Broken Back (Fractured Spine)

Causes: Fractures and dislocations of the spinal column are usually the result of some traumatic incident (e.g., an auto accident, a fall, or a blow with a stick across the back).

Symptoms: Generally, if the cat has been involved in an accident and cannot move both back legs, and there is no response when the toe is firmly pinched, it is logical to assume that the animal has a break or fracture of the spine. The cat usually lies with its front legs extended, and is insensitive to pain below the affected portion of the spine. Urinary and fecal incontinence or retention are present.

The above symptoms could also indicate a slipped disk. But the slipped disk occurs spontaneously, not as the result of a traumatic incident.

Treatment: If the cat has been hit by a car, do not move it unless absolutely necessary. Telephone a vet, the police, or the A.S.P.C.A. If the animal must be moved, wrap the cat in a blanket or coat and carry it to the vet in a basket or box.

Prognosis: The prognosis for cats that suffer fractures and dislocations of the spine is not very hopeful. In the majority of cases, the animal will have to be put to sleep.

Broken Tail

Fractures of the tail occur during accidents, and in cats confined to small areas. It usually takes about two weeks for a tail fracture to heal.

Fractures at root of tail: If the break occurs at the root of the tail, the full length of the tail will hang straight down. There will be pain and swelling at the fracture site.

Treatment: The owner should not attempt to treat root fractures. Professional assistance is necessary. If the cat is in pain, administer one-half of a 250-mg. Tylenol ® tablet, then take the cat to a veterinarian. (See How to Administer Tablets and Pills.)

Fractures along length of tail: Fractures of this type are easily identifiable: the cat can move its tail up to the fracture site, while the portion of the tail beyond the fracture hangs limply.

Treatment: Should there be a delay of more than twenty-four hours before the cat can be seen by a vet, apply adhesive tape to support the length of the damaged tail. Tape the break tightly enough to provide support but not so tight that the circulation is cut off.

Fractures of tip of tail: Wrap adhesive tape around the fracture; be careful not to tape it too tightly. It usually takes about two weeks for a tail fracture to heal.

Treatment: Cats with fractures, or suspected fractures, of the tail should be examined by a vet. Nerve damage often results, and that portion of the tail beyond the fracture may then have to be removed surgically.

Fractured Spine (See Broken Back)

Slipped Disk

A painful abnormality of the spine that is very rare in cats.

Causes: Accidents; obesity; spontaneous prolapse.

Symptoms: Acute pain when the cat attempts to walk. In some cases, the cat cannot move its back legs.

There may be rigidity or tenseness of the abdomen. Touch the cat's stomach lightly: the skin may be as tight as a drum. There may be retention of urine and feces at first. Then, as the bladder and the small intestine fill up, the cat is unable to control itself and involuntary passage of body wastes results.

Treatment: To ease the cat's pain, administer analgesics. (See Analgesics.) While most mild cases of slipped disk will right themselves, if the condition persists or recurs, surgery may be necessary. Consult a veterinarian.

10

Problems Affecting
the Whole Body

Allergy: General (See Asthma, Eczema, Hay Fever, Hives)

An allergy is a reaction by the body to a specific substance to which it has become oversensitized by previous exposure.

Causes: Hair of other animals; pollen; drugs; certain foods; detergents; fleas. Individual animals vary in their sensitivity to these causes.

Symptoms: Vomiting; diarrhea; running eyes; red and itching skin; swollen lips and eyelids. While these symptoms are present in other disease states, they will be accompanied by additional symptoms. When they appear on their own, for no obvious reason, suspect an allergy.

Treatment: The best way of treating an allergy is to remove the cause. Where this is not possible, either because the allergic substance cannot be identified or because it is in the air (e.g., pollen), it may be necessary to consult a veterinarian, who will probably administer antihistamines and corticosteroids. The cat owner should be aware that this is professional treatment and that the indiscriminate use of these or any drugs is very dangerous. Further, the use of human medication in the treatment of animals is doubly dangerous, since strength and dosage vary greatly.

Anemia

A blood condition in which the oxygen-carrying capacity of the blood is reduced.

Causes: Loss of blood; blood destruction due to infection (e.g., feline infectious anemia, microscopic blood parasites); poor blood formation (iron deficiency).

Symptoms: Lethargy; rapid pulse; unnatural paleness around the eyes, nose, and gums. (See Taking the Pulse.)

To some extent, the symptoms vary from one case to another. A cat suffering from a debilitating disease will develop this pallor gradually, while a cat that has a hemorrhaging gastric ulcer or one involved in a car accident will suddenly become very pale around the mucous membranes. A cat with feline infectious anemia will have a temperature that fluctuates from normal to very high. (See Taking Temperature.)

Treatment: Since anemia is almost always symptomatic of other diseases or deficiencies, all anemic animals require professional treatment. In chronic anemia, if professional help is not immediately available administer one-half of a 30-mg. ferrous sulfate tablet once a day. (See How to Administer Tablets and Pills.) Consult a vet for further treatment.

Calcium Deficiency

The main function of calcium in the diet is to aid the growth and formation of teeth and bones. Proper amounts of calcium in the diet of kittens are essential. A lack of calcium in the diet will cause rickets, resulting in swollen tender joints, arched back, and stiff legs. Acute calcium deficiency in the lactating cat will produce a condition called milk fever. (See Milk Fever.)

Treatment: Although milk is a natural source of calcium, a cat suffering from a calcium deficiency needs a concentrated dose. Prepare a solution made with 1 teaspoon of calcium gluconate powder (available at drugstores) added to 10 teaspoons of water. Shake until powder is dissolved. Since the cat will probably refuse to drink this voluntarily, the owner should be prepared to force-feed. (See Force-Feeding.) A convulsing cat should receive intravenous calcium.

Diabetes Insipidus (Drinking Diabetes)

Symptoms: Increased thirst (be sure to keep the cat's water bowl full); frequent, pale-colored urination. Laboratory tests will show no sugar in the urine. There is no smell of acetone on the breath as in diabetes mellitus. (See also Chronic Interstitial Nephritis.)

Treatment: Your vet may put your cat on a course of hormone treatment.

Nursing diabetic cats: The diabetic cat requires a diet that is high in protein and low in carbohydrates. Fortunately, most canned animal foods provide adequate nourishment when supplemented by two raw eggs a week mixed into the cat's food, to supply the necessary amount of fat. Diabetic cats should not be fed dry pet foods.

Diabetes Mellitus (Sugar Diabetes)

Cause: Diabetes is a chronic disorder in which there is an abnormal amount of sugar in the blood and urine due to a malfunctioning of the pancreas. This condition is rare in cats.

Symptoms: Increased appetite; increased thirst; frequent urination; weight loss; traces of sugar in the urine; a sweetish odor of acetone (smells like nail polish remover) on the cat's breath. (See Bad Breath.) Secondary symptoms of cataracts may appear in the eyes. If left untreated, the animal will fall into a diabetic coma. (See Unconsciousness.)

Collecting urine sample: A definite diagnosis must be made by a vet, after analysis of a urine sample. The simplest way to collect a sample is to put a handful of sand in one end of the cat's litter tray. Place a block under that end of the tray, so that it stands a few inches off the ground. The urine will filter through the sand and collect at the lower end. Only a few drops are needed for an analysis. (See Taking Samples of Feces and Urine.)

Treatment: Home treatment, after professional consultation, may consist of daily injections of insulin. (See How to Give an Injection.) The drug should always be given before feeding.

Overdose: If an accidental overdose of insulin is administered, insulin coma will follow. This condition can be reversed by giving a tablespoon of dextrose monohydrate or a tablespoon of crushed or powdered sugar. Sprinkle a little at a time into the unconscious cat's mouth.

Distemper (Enteritis)

A very common, serious, and highly contagious viral disease.

Symptoms: Depression and lethargy; loss of appetite; high temperature (101.5-106°F.); vomiting; dehydration. To test for dehydration, pinch a bit of the cat's skin between your fingers: the skin remains raised for a few minutes instead of resuming its normal shape. A classic symptom of this disease is that of a cat sitting hunched over its drinking bowl without drinking.

Treatment: If any combination of the above symptoms appears, seek professional help at once. Feline distemper develops rapidly and can kill a cat within eight hours from the onset of initial symptoms.

Prevention: All cats should be vaccinated against feline distemper. Kittens may be vaccinated any time after weaning at eight to ten weeks of age, with a booster shot once a year. (See Vaccination.) If you aren't sure whether your cat has been vaccinated, have it done again.

Drowning

Although cats (despite their aversion to water) are

usually excellent swimmers, like human swimmers they can also drown.

Treatment: Get the cat out of the water. If the animal is unconscious, lay it on its side and open its mouth. Make sure that its tongue is out and that there is no obstruction in the windpipe. Use your finger to check for grass, sand, mud, etc., in the cat's mouth.

If the cat remains unconscious, lift it by its hind legs and allow the water to drain out of its mouth. Administer artificial respiration or mouth-to-nostril resuscitation, which is slightly more effective. Hold the cat's mouth closed with cupped hands and blow down its nose until its chest fills up. Let the chest empty naturally. Repeat every five seconds. (See also Artificial Respiration.)

Electric Shock

Cause: Chewing on an electric cord. So if you find your cat lying unconscious next to a badly frayed electric cord, that's it!

Warning: Often a shocked cat will urinate and the pool of urine is an excellent electrical conductor. Do not step in the urine, and do not touch the cat until you have turned off the current, or you will need someone to give *you* first aid.

If you are unable to turn off the electricity, put on a rubber glove or grab a thick, dry towel and pull the electric plug out of the outlet. Or, use a broom to push the animal out of the urine and away from the electric cord.

Treatment: If the cat has not regained consciousness by this time, administer artificial respiration. (See *Swinging technique* under Artificial Respiration.) When the cat comes to, treat for shock. (See Shock.)

Excessive Thirst (Drink-Vomit Cycle)

Symptoms: Increased thirst is a symptom of several conditions, all of them serious. (See *Note* below.) Since the average cat owner is not competent to make a diagnosis, follow these general rules until a vet can examine the cat.

Treatment: Never withhold water from a cat with excessive thirst, unless the cat is vomiting. When a cat starts on the drink-vomit cycle, it will continue drinking and then vomiting until dehydration and death occur.

To break this cycle, withhold all water for twelve hours. Then feed the cat 1 tablespoon of a water and dextrose monohydrate mixture, every two hours for twelve hours. The mixture should consist of 3–4 tablespoons of dextrose monohydrate dissolved in 1 pint of water. (While cats will not usually drink such a sweet mixture willingly, a cat that has not had a drink for twelve hours will drink almost anything.) An ice cube put in the animal's drinking bowl may also be given every hour, so that the cat can lick the cube for the moisture.

If the cat is still vomiting after twelve hours, seek professional help.

Note (differential diagnoses): Diabetes; chronic interstitial nephritis; pyometritis; increased body temperature; poisoning; enteritis; gastritis; other infections. These disease states are really beyond the normal scope of home treatment. They are noted here to impress the pet owner with the seriousness of the excessive thirst symptom. A cat exhibiting symptoms of excessive thirst must be carefully observed for a few hours; if the symptoms are confirmed, professional help is necessary.

Fits, Convulsions

Causes: The cause of a fit cannot be diagnosed from the type of fit or its severity. A number of agents, ranging from teething problems to serious infections to poisons such as strychnine, may cause fits.

Symptoms: Fits take several forms, all of them violent and frightening. The fit usually begins with the cat shaking its head. This is followed by champing of the jaws, salivation, incoordination, screaming, and the involuntary passage of urine and feces. The cat may then fall on its side and make running movements. The action of the jaws converts the saliva into a viscid froth, causing the cat to foam at the mouth and often terrifying those who should be helping the animal.

Treatment: The only thing you can do for a cat that is having a fit is prevent the cat from hurting itself. First, make sure that it does not hurt you. Remember, the most affectionate pet becomes a dangerous animal during a fit. Do not try to calm it by petting or stroking. It will not do your cat any good. It will just get you bitten or scratched. Don't waste time talking to the cat; it cannot hear you.

Move the cat into a place where it cannot injure itself. (See below for technique.) Get some blankets or pillows and throw them into a closet or small room without furniture or sharp corners. If possible, darken the room.

Technique for moving a cat: Throw a blanket or coat over the cat and carry it in this to the room or closet. Once the cat is in the safe room, leave it alone. The fit will pass. It may take five minutes, it could take thirty, but eventually the fit should pass. When it does, allow the cat to rest quietly. Seek professional help.

The fit may have been caused by epilepsy, a virus, worms, teething, or be the sequel to a very high fever. In young kittens, the cause may be something as simple as overexcitement. (See also Rabies.) Further treatment will depend upon the cause of the fit. Without medical training, one can only make a guess, not a diagnosis.

Remember, all you can do is to deal with the immediate situation. Prevent the animal from hurting itself. Further treatment must be left to your veterinarian.

FRACTURES

Fracture is the term used to describe a broken bone.

Simple fracture: If only the bone is broken and there is no communicating wound between the fracture and the skin, it is called a simple fracture.

Compound fracture: If the skin over the fracture site is broken, making it possible for germs to enter from the external wound, it is called a compound fracture. In this condition, the bone protrudes through the skin.

Complicated fracture: This type of fracture may be either simple or compound, but there is also injury to some internal organ, blood vessel, nerve, or joint.

An originally simple fracture can be turned into a compound or complicated fracture by allowing the injured cat complete freedom of movement, or by carelessness or ignorance on the part of the owner.

When rendering first aid for fractures, there are two main objectives: guarding against further injury, and reducing the animal's pain.

Causes: Most fractures are caused by accidents; they also occur spontaneously when a bone is undergoing pathological change (e.g., in calcium deficiency or in bone cancer).

General treatment: Injured cats must be approached and handled with great caution. An animal in pain is dangerous to its owner and itself. If a fracture is suspected, handle the limb or broken bone as little as possible. Make the cat as comfortable and as warm as possible. Administer one-half of a 250-mg. Tylenol ® tablet once only, to control the pain. (See How to Administer Tablets and Pills.)

Basic first aid is aimed at providing a support for the fractured bone. To accomplish this a splint is applied to the fractured bone, at the point of the fracture. The splint serves as a temporary support between which the broken bones are held in place until professional help can be obtained. (See instructions for making a splint under Fractures of the Limbs.)

Do not attempt to reduce fractures and to reset broken bones. This will cause extreme pain and should be done only under anesthetic. Seek professional assistance as soon as possible.

Fractures of the Bones of the Foot

If the cat is acutely lame, and no swelling is visible, it is fair to assume that the bone is damaged and, quite possibly, fractured.

Treatment: Put bits of cotton between the cat's toes and wrap an Ace ® bandage around the leg. Cover the bandage with surgical tape to keep it in place. (See Bandaging the Leg.) Seek professional help.

Fractures of the Jaws

Fractures of the jaws are frequently seen in cats that have fallen from a considerable height: the front legs give way and the chin hits the ground, causing a fracture of the lower jaw. In lower jaw fractures, the jaw usually hangs slightly open and there is profuse salivation, dribbling, and drooling.

If the cat falls from an even greater height, there may be a fracture of the upper jaw which, under close examination, appears as a split in the roof of the mouth or a pronounced split or displacement of the front teeth.

Treatment: Upper or lower jaw, the difference is academic: there is no effective home treatment for this condition. Once you have determined that the cat has a fractured jaw, get the injured animal to a vet immediately. Although many fractures will heal by themselves, there is the very real danger of the jaw healing improperly.

Fractures of the Limbs

The fractures most commonly seen in cats are fractures involving the legs.

Symptoms: Acute and profound lameness of the affected leg; considerable pain; possible swelling; possible shortening. When the cat is lifted off the ground, the affected limb will swing freely. Generally, some or all of these symptoms can be seen in a cat with a leg fracture.

Fractures of the upper parts of the limbs: These are

extremely difficult to splint and should be left alone until professional help is available.

Fractures of the lower parts of the limbs: These are among the most common fractures seen. The cat will be unable to put its injured foot on the ground and, as it hobbles along, the leg will swing freely. If professional help is not available within twenty-four hours, fractures of the lower leg should be supported by a simple splint.

To make a splint: Lay the cat on its side, injured leg uppermost. Then place the injured leg on a thin piece of wood or corrugated cardboard, and tape the leg to the wood with strips of adhesive tape.

Have an assistant hold the cat by its scruff with one hand, and with the other hand hold the injured leg on the splint while you tape the leg to the splint. This splint is intended simply to prevent excessive movement and not as a permanent repair or as a substitute for the services of a veterinarian.

Fractures of the Pelvis

A cat with a fractured pelvis will be unable to support any weight on either of its hind legs. However, since a cat with both hind legs fractured or a spinal fracture will also be unable to stand, X ray is the only definite means of diagnosing a fractured pelvis.

Treatment: A fracture of the pelvis does not require splinting. Keep the cat in a confined space. Consult a vet.

Fractures of the Skull

Seen after road accidents, falls, blows; may cause unconsciousness, nosebleeds, and incoordination.

Treatment: Skull fracture can be diagnosed only by X-ray. If a fracture of the skull is suspected, do not bandage the skull; it may be a depressed fracture, and bandaging would only make it worse. If there is bleeding, use simple first aid to stop it. Be very gentle. Give no drugs or fluids until a vet has been consulted.

Gangrene

The term *gangrene* applies to either a specific localized infection, or a part of the body in which the tissues are dead because of restricted blood supply to that part.

Infection: When gangrene in the cat is due to an infection, it is usually the result of bite wounds, especially on the feet. If the infection is left untreated, it may become gangrenous. A bite around the wrist area can become infected, causing swelling and pus that block the blood vessels leading to the toes and resulting in gangrene of the toes.

The infection develops within two or three days; the infected area becomes swollen, foul-smelling, and gives off a bubbly discharge.

Treatment: Consult a veterinarian immediately.

Blood restriction: Gangrene caused by restriction of blood supply to a part of the body is seen when bandages are applied too tightly or when a tourniquet is left on too long. Gangrene sets in, affecting the surrounding area. It also occurs (too frequently) when children put rubber bands around the cat's paws or scrotum.

Treatment: Remove the source of constriction. Clean the area with pHisoDerm ® or soap and water. Apply warm compresses to encourage the blood to circulate again. Get professional help.

Grass Seeds

In the summer and early autumn, drying grass seeds can cause a good deal of pain by penetrating between the cat's toes, or into its ears or eyes. If left untreated, the seeds, which are barbed like fishhooks, will migrate inward, eventually producing pus-discharging wounds.

In the ears: A grass seed in the ear causes very painful symptoms. The cat rubs its face on the ground, paws at its ears, and walks with its head on one side as though attempting to dislodge something.

Treatment: Pour warm olive oil or cooking oil into the ear; massage gently to float the seeds out.

In the eyes: Profuse crying from one eye only; becomes very red and obviously painful.

Treatment: If the seed has not penetrated the eyeball, wash it out of the eye with a saline solution. (See Saline Solution.) If it has penetrated the eyeball, do not attempt to remove it. Take the cat to the vet. Determining whether the seed has penetrated the eyeball is a matter of observation. With the aid of a flashlight you will be able to see if there is something protruding from the cat's eyeball.

Between the toes: A grass seed lodged between the toes produces pustules that may cause the cat to limp. If left untreated, the seed will work its way into the foot, producing breaks in the skin.

Treatment: If you can see the seed, use a pair of tweezers to pull it out.

Growths, Tumors, Cancers

Tumors or cancers can affect any organ, system, or part of the cat's body at any age. They are divided into two groups: benign and malignant.

Benign tumors: Grow slowly; clearly defined, round lumps; cool to the touch; do not spread.

Malignant tumors: Grow rapidly; not clearly defined (sometimes it is difficult to tell where the tumor ends and the healthy part of the body begins); warm to the touch; tend to ulcerate; spread to other parts of the body. If left untreated, they eventually cause death.

Treatment: Since any swelling may be a tumor, it should be examined immediately by a vet. Even a malignant tumor can be controlled if it is caught early.

Heat Stroke

Causes: Prolonged exposure to a source of heat or overcrowding. Classic cases of heat stroke occur when cats are packed into traveling cages that are too small and improperly ventilated. The condition is more common in cats with heavy coats, and is aggravated by lack of water.

Symptoms: Early stages—panting; dullness; stumbling;

sweating through the foot pads. *Later stages*—very high fever (up to 110°F.); coma; death.

Treatment: Give the cat water immediately. Cool the animal by hosing or sponging with cold water and by applying ice packs all over its body, with special attention to the head and chest. Give the cat a bowlful of water, with 1 tablespoon of glucose mixed in. Allow the animal time to rest and drink. High fever should not be lowered too quickly. Check rectal temperature every five minutes. (See Taking Temperature.)

Lightning

Although it occurs rarely, cats taking shelter under trees or in close contact with metallic objects are occasionally struck by lightning.

Symptoms: Cat may be burned; may show signs of shock (See Shock); incoordination or even paralysis.

Treatment: Treat for shock by keeping the cat warm and quiet; then treat the burns. (See Burns.) Administer up to one cup of a simple stimulant (e.g., cooled tea or black coffee). Hold the cat in a semi-upright position; pour the fluid down its throat slowly, a little at a time, to prevent the animal from choking. Get professional help.

Motion Sickness (Airsickness, Car Sickness, Seasickness)

A common condition in cats.

Symptoms: Restlessness; excessive salivation; persistent vomiting.

Treatment: Before the trip, administer an animal tranquilizer (can be obtained from the vet). It is never a good idea to give a cat a tranquilizer intended for human consumption, since there is a vast difference in proper dosage. In extraordinary circumstances, if animal tranquilizers are not available, preparations for human travel sickness (e.g., Dramamine ®, available at drugstores) may be administered orally. Exact dosage depends on the size of the animal.

Prevention: Withhold all food for twelve hours before long journeys, but give your cat plenty of water. To prevent car sickness, get your cat accustomed to car travel by taking it on short trips whenever possible. Allow the cat to spend time in the car when it is not in use.

Neuralgia

Cause: Nerve pain.

Symptoms: Sudden and obvious pain; tense muscles in the cat's neck, back, or legs. Attacks of neuralgia are intermittent and may last for several hours.

Treatment: Keep the cat warm and allow it to rest. An infrared lamp is a great comfort to a cat suffering from neuralgia. Mount the lamp about three feet above the cat's bed and leave it on all night. In the absence of such a lamp, an electric blanket, hot water bottle, or heating pad is helpful. (Special heating pads are now available for pets.) Administer one-half of a 250-mg. Tylenol ® tablet. (See How to Administer Tablets and Pills.) Do not repeat dosage for seventy-two hours.

Pain

Symptoms: There is no register for pain. The cat owner must observe the animal's reactions as a guide to the location and severity of the pain. Cats show pain by assuming an abnormal position or by abnormal behavior.

Pain in different parts of the body produces different reactions. For example: pain in the legs produces lameness; pain in the abdomen causes restlessness, sitting or lying in abnormal positions, and whining. There is also a tendency to seek out cold places, such as cement floors, to lie on. Pain in the head produces languor. The cat paws at its head, is restless, and may press its head against the wall. Acute pain causes the cat to cry, meow, whimper, and act frightened. The cat will look at or lick the affected area.

A cat manifesting symptoms of pain should be carefully observed. Its behavior may give you a clue to the problem: a cat with a foreign body in its paw will chew at its foot; a cat with a foreign body in its mouth will paw at its mouth.

Rabies

Although rabies, a viral infection, usually occurs in bats, dogs, foxes, and skunks, all warm-blooded animals—including man and cats—are susceptible.

Cause: Transmitted by an infected animal biting another animal. The incubation period varies from fifteen days to several months.

Symptoms: The symptoms of rabies are easily confused with those of many other diseases. They include: a marked change in behavior (e.g., docile cats become aggressive, aggressive cats docile); vomiting; diarrhea. The cat often behaves as if it has a foreign body in its mouth; coughing, drooling, and pawing at its mouth. From one to three days after the onset of these symptoms, the affected cat will become vicious, biting and scratching at the slightest provocation. In the final stages, many cats that are normally quite sociable will seek solitude.

Treatment: Treatment is given to any human being who may have been bitten. If one has been exposed to a cat who is suspected of being rabid, the animal should be confined but not killed, in order for a correct diagnosis to be made. If you are bitten by any stray animal, or if rabies is suspected, call a doctor at once.

Prevention: Beware of all strays. Have your cat vaccinated against rabies. If you have the slightest suspicion that your cat may be rabid, confine the cat and notify your veterinarian.

Shock

Shock is the term used to describe a state of collapse characterized by an acute and progressive failure of the circulatory system.

Causes: While the exact causes of shock are unknown, the condition results from severe trauma caused by serious injuries, massive hemorrhage, heart failure, serious burns, anemia, and dehydration.

Symptoms: Apathy; low temperature; pale gums and tongue; rapid, thready pulse; rapid, shallow breathing; thirst; and, finally, complete collapse.

Treatment: Keep the cat warm by wrapping it in a blanket. Keep the animal as quiet as possible. Take it to a veterinarian immediately. The treatment of choice is to restore the amount of circulating fluid in the blood vessels by means of transfusion.

Trembling, Shivering

Causes: Cats shiver when they are frightened, cold, running a high fever, or overexcited. Frightened cats will also pant.

Treatment: Shivering or trembling that goes on for longer than half an hour is a sign that something is seriously wrong. Examine the cat for fever. (See Taking Temperature.)

Unconsciousness

When you find a cat unconscious, unless the cause is immediately apparent (e.g., a large gaping wound), do not waste time looking for the reason. The only exception to this is when the animal has been in contact with an electric cord. (See Electric Shock.)

Causes: The reasons that cats lose consciousness may be divided into two very general categories: primary and secondary causes.

Primary causes: Result of a lesion (break) affecting the nervous system and the brain. This occurs after car accidents or similar injuries, fits, strokes, and narcosis produced by poisoning.

Secondary causes: Result of ailments affecting other areas of the body: diabetic coma, uremic coma (poison from the kidneys), calcium deficiency, shock, electric shock, drowning, and heart attack.

Treatment: If the cat does not appear to be breathing, do not assume that it is dead, unless certain other symptoms are evident (e.g., dilated pupils; cold, stiff body; no heartbeat or pulse). Even if you think the cat is dead and you cannot detect breathing, give artificial respiration for at least thirty minutes unless rigor mortis is evident. (See Artificial Respiration.)

Fainting: Cats faint if the blood supply to the brain is reduced or is deficient in oxygen. This occurs in cats that are in a state of shock, or whose hearts are not functioning properly.

Treatment: Cats that have fainted will recover spontaneously. Most cats recover from faints in three to four minutes. Make sure the animal's tongue is out, and that nothing is blocking the windpipe.

Vomiting

Causes: Infectious disease (e.g., feline enteritis); acute abdomen (e.g., peritonitis, intestinal obstruction); indigestion (e.g., overeating); metabolic disorders (e.g., hepatitis, nephritis); drugs (e.g., digitalis); nervous disorders (e.g., motion sickness, fear); pharyngeal irritation (e.g., tonsillitis); poisoning; parasites (e.g., tapeworm); hernias; tumors; inflammation of the gullet.

Warning: Do not administer emetics to an animal that is vomiting.

Blood in Vomit

Causes: Fresh blood in your cat's vomit may be caused by accidents, tumors, or foreign bodies that have cut the mouth, throat, or gullet. If the blood is black, it comes from the stomach or from the small intestine, and may be caused by a stomach ulcer or by tumors.

Treatment: There is no home treatment for this condition, since it is not possible for the cat owner to diagnose the cause accurately. As a temporary measure, the cat should not be fed. Consult a vet immediately.

Drink-Vomit Cycle (See Excessive Thirst)

Vomiting Induced by Poisons

The group of poisons that cause vomiting includes most of the common poisons (e.g., arsenic, phosphorus, and decayed foods).

Symptoms: Burns in cat's mouth or on its tongue; vomit has strong acid odor.

Treatment: Administer either 2 tablespoons of corn oil or a solution made by adding 3 tablespoons of sodium bicarbonate to ½ pint of water, to soothe the stomach lining. (See Force-Feeding.)

WEIGHT PROBLEMS

Excessive Appetite

Causes: A dramatic increase in appetite suggests: abdominal tumors; diseases that interfere with food absorption; fat deposits common in spayed queens and neutered tomcats; simple greed (may be due to a neurotic condition or to brain damage); pregnancy.

Treatment: Depends upon the cause. Abdominal tumors and food absorption diseases require professional treatment. In the case of desexed cats, feed them less than they want. Simple greed is beyond the scope of treatment, and the last cause treats itself.

Loss of Appetite (Anorexia)

It is not unusual for a cat to neglect its food for twenty-four hours. But if the cat refuses food after that length of time, consider this loss of appetite as a symptom of something else.

Causes: (1) Generalized disease. The cat acts and looks ill. It may be apathetic, listless, feverish, its coat may be dull. These are very general symptoms, and are a good reason why cat owners should observe their cats while in good health. Deviation from the norm is easy to recognize for those familiar with their pet's normal behavior and appearance. (2) Tartar on the teeth. This can cause pain when chewing. (3) Foreign body in the mouth (e.g., a splinter of bone between the teeth). (4) Sore mouth or sore throat.

Treatment: Examine the cat's mouth with a flashlight, checking for sores, tartar, inflammation, and obstructions.

(1) Loss of appetite due to a generalized disease must be treated by a vet. (2) If the cat's teeth reveal an accumulation of tartar, see Tartar on the Teeth for a description of the treatment of this condition. (3) If a foreign body is in the mouth, open the cat's mouth and remove the object. (See How to Open a Cat's Mouth.) (4) To check for a sore throat, gently feel around the cat's larynx. If the throat is sore, the cat will cough. Consult a vet. If none of the above are observed, take the cat's temperature. If it is above normal, consult a vet. (See Taking Temperature.)

If there does not seem to be anything wrong with the cat, but it still refuses to eat, try to tempt it with a change of diet. Try succulent taste treats (e.g., boiled deboned chicken, strong cheeses, tuna fish, or meat extracts). Cats will not eat food that they cannot smell, so when a cat refuses to eat, it's wise to check for cat flu symptoms. (See Flu.)

Weight Gain

Causes: A great increase in weight over a three to four week period is abnormal and suggests one of the following possibilities: abdominal tumor (see Index); fluid in the abdomen (some serious diseases produce large amounts of fluid in the abdomen); compulsive eating (may be the result of simple greed or brain damage); pregnancy; tendency of desexed cats to put on weight; thyroid deficiency.

Treatment: This list is a general guide to the possible causes of a sudden weight increase in your cat. Proper diagnosis and treatment must be left to a vet.

Weight Loss

Causes: A sudden loss in weight may be caused by: reduced intake of food; persistent vomiting; reduced absorption of food due to disease states (e.g., chronic nephritis, hepatitis); tumors; parasites.

Treatment: Although you may not be able to cure the ailment, if you can identify the cause, you may be able to treat the secondary symptoms as they arise. If there is drastic weight loss, do not wait until the cat is down to fur and bones before you get professional assistance.

11

Problems of Female Cats Only

Abortion or Miscarriage

Miscarriage, or abortion, occurs when the fetus is expelled from the uterus before the end of the normal gestation period (sixty-three to sixty-five days).

Causes: Miscarriage is infrequent among cats, but does occur as the result of infection, hormonal imbalance, accident, or poor feeding.

Early symptoms: As the birth process begins, the pregnant cat will show signs of discomfort and restlessness, accompanied by bleeding and, later, a clear discharge from the vulva. Since the embryos are small and soft, the miscarriage that follows is usually rapid and painless.

Treatment: Try to stanch the bleeding by applying an absorbent pad to the vagina. Keep the animal calm and quiet. Get professional help without delay.

Emergencies: In some rare instances, severe hemorrhaging may occur during or immediately after the birth. *This is an emergency.*

Agalactia (Inability to Give Milk)

Agalactia is the inability of the mother cat to give milk. It often occurs in cats giving birth to their first litter, especially in oriental breeds.

Causes: The cause may be hereditary, the result of hormonal imbalance, or the sequel to an infection or breast cancer.

Symptoms: The behavior of the kittens is the best indication of agalactia. If the kittens are not getting their milk, they will be restless and fretful, just as a human baby would be. The mother, however, will appear quite normal.

Treatment: Apply warm compresses to the mother's mammary glands for ten minutes at a time, four to five times a day. Gently massage the mammary glands with olive oil to stimulate and restore their function. Consult a veterinarian about hormone therapy with pituitary hormones. This treatment may induce milk production within twenty-four hours.

Treatment of agalactia, of course, applies only to the mother. Meanwhile, the newborn kittens, awaiting the production of milk, must be fed every two hours. (See Orphan Kittens.)

Birth

Generally, birth occurs sixty-three to sixty-five days after conception, though occasionally a queen may give birth up to a week early or a week late. While it isn't necessary to have a veterinarian present at the birth, it is sensible to have the pregnant cat examined by a vet prior to the event. Although cats are quite expert at home delivery, it is a good idea to observe the birth from the sidelines in case something does go wrong. Keep the vet's telephone number handy.

Signs of approaching birth: Approximately six hours before birth, the mother becomes restless and begins preparing a place to give birth (usually the most inconvenient place!). Vomiting may occur. The cat's body temperature drops three degrees to about 98°F. The vulva becomes enlarged and pinkish. The pelvic ligaments slacken, causing some loss of coordination in the hind legs.

Stages of labor: Within an hour before birth, the mother grows increasingly nervous and may start glancing at her flanks. Occasional contractions of the abdomen become more frequent.

The queen lies down as the contractions become more frequent. As the fetus enters the pelvis, there is definite straining. The water bag, which looks like a black grape, appears at the vulva. The queen licks the water bag to rupture it. After the water breaks, the kittens, each in its own sac, will begin to appear, protruding from the vulva.

After violent expulsive efforts by the mother, the infant animal is born. Often the mother will cry out as the kitten's head comes through. In a normal birth, the interval between kittens is generally from five to thirty minutes. The final stage is the expulsion of the remaining membranes from the cat's womb. This can occur as long as one hour after the kittens have been born.

Complications: If there is more than a two–minute delay after the head and front legs are out, the kitten should be gently pulled out. Use a towel to grip without slipping and pull only during a contraction. Grip as high as you can. It is essential that the kitten should be extracted as quickly and as carefully as possible.

Some kittens are born head first, some are born tail first. Both positions are normal, but if the kitten is born tail first it should come out fairly rapidly after the water has broken. If the kitten is not out within ten minutes, telephone the vet. If the kitten is born with the membranes surrounding it still intact, remove them rapidly, if the mother does not do so. Do not immediately discard the sacs and placentas as the mother cat should eat some of the placenta.

Every kitten should be checked immediately to be sure that its mouth is free of mucus, enabling it to breathe freely. If breathing does not occur at once, rub the kitten briskly with a clean, rough towel. If this does not work, try mouth-to-nostril breathing by blowing into the kitten's nose. Or place the kitten in a bowl of warm water and then plunge it into a bowl of cold water. Once breathing has begun, put the kitten back with its mother and let her lick it dry.

Umbilical cord: The umbilical cord should break when the kitten comes out of the membrane. If it does not, tie the cord off with clean, boiled thread, two inches from the kitten, and cut it on the side of the knot farthest away from the kitten.

Afterbirth: After the kittens are born, more membranes may be expelled. A greenish black discharge, several hours after birth, is quite normal.

The size of a normal litter varies from one to six kittens.

If a queen seems nervous or overprotective towards her newly born litter, or if she objects to strangers or even family handling her young, humor her. Keep the strangers and the rest of the family away from the kittens. Of course, children are usually the main offenders, and it is difficult to refuse them the delights of handling newly born kittens, but if the kittens' mother shows any resentment, this must be done. After all, they are *her* kittens.

Diet for Brood Queen

A brood queen is a cat that is used for breeding. Brood queens may be fed their usual diet with extra milk and fat added. An extra half pint of milk per day plus two egg yolks should be adequate. Also add 2 tablespoons of calcium gluconate (available at drugstores) once a week to the queen's food.

Do not feed the queen dried foods from the day of mating until birth occurs. These contain carbohydrates, which tend to make cats fatter, and a pregnant animal should not be overweight.

Heat Periods (Estrous Cycle)

The heat, or breeding, period (estrous cycle) takes place twice a year, usually in spring and early fall, and lasts for about four weeks. During these weeks, the queen comes into heat several times, each heat lasting for five to ten days.

The first heat period occurs when the queen is six to fifteen months old. After giving birth, the first heat usually occurs within four to five weeks.

Symptoms: A cat in heat is a most distressing sight to the inexperienced owner. The queen rolls about on the floor, her back flat, hindquarters and tail raised. She yowls loudly and persistently and performs pedaling movements with her back legs.

Treatment: A male cat, or a set of earplugs (for yourself). If you do not want kittens, keep the queen indoors during her heat. She is not in agony; she just looks that way.

Hemorrhage from the Vagina

While very slight bleeding from the vagina is normal during heat periods, heavy bleeding requires the immediate assistance of a veterinarian.

Treatment: Keep the queen warm and quiet until professional help is available. (See Shock; Abortion or Miscarriage; Pyometra.)

Mating

Queens should not be permitted to mate until they are at least nine months old. The gestation period is sixty-three to sixty-five days. Tomcats usually begin mating at six to eight months of age.

Queens have two or three breeding seasons per year and

three or four heats during these seasons. A queen can, and if given the opportunity will, mate again when her kittens are about six weeks old.

Since the average queen can produce as many as three to four litters a year, the question of whether to have a queen spayed is of some relevance to conscientious cat owners.

The best age to have a cat desexed is from four to five months for females and six months for males.

Milk Fever (Eclampsia)

This serious condition may occur in queens which have just had large litters.

Cause: Calcium deficiency.

Symptoms: Milk fever usually manifests itself just before the kittens are weaned—about five to six weeks after birth. The queen becomes very restless. She meows a great deal and lies with her legs extended, breathing rapidly. She may lose her sense of coordination and fall over when she tries to stand. This stage is associated with a rise in body temperature, above 103°F.; there is drooling, rigidity, and convulsions.

Warning: Do not allow the queen's symptoms to progress. If she is in this state and left untreated, she will die.

Treatment: Treatment is simple, but it must be administered by a veterinarian. It consists of calcium gluconate administered intravenously. If convulsions have not started, the owner can mix 4 ounces of calcium gluconate with 1 pint of water and give the solution orally until the symptoms stop or the cat can be taken to the vet. (See Force-Feeding.)

Prevention: During lactation, give the queen plenty of milk with bone-meal crackers crumbled in it and add calcium gluconate powder to her food. Feed one-half teaspoon daily.

Mother Cat Eating Her Kittens

A queen having her first litter should be carefully watched; in certain circumstances, she may attempt to eat her young. This is not as monstrous or as abnormal as it sounds. It may be the result of a natural fright response. More often, however, it is caused by a faulty placenta-eating instinct. In this case, the mother simply does not know where the placenta (afterbirth) ends and her newborn kittens begin.

Nipple Soreness (See Agalactia)

Cause: This condition, often encountered in a mother cat who is nursing her litter, is caused by the nails of the kittens pricking the soft flesh of the queen's teats.

Symptoms: The kittens scream for food; the queen's nipples are red and cracked.

Treatment: If the nipples are sore and red, apply Vaseline® twice a day. Rub it in well, and remove surplus with cotton. If the nipples have become cracked, bathe them three times a day in a solution of ½ teaspoon of boric acid added to 1 cup of water. After bathing, dry the nipples gently but thoroughly with cotton; apply Vaseline®.

Prevention: The nails of kittens should not be clipped or cut; they should be filed once a week.

Postpuerperal Metritis

Causes: This is an acute infection of the womb that may result from injury or infection during the delivery of kittens.

Symptoms: An abnormal, dark, bloody vaginal discharge occurs two to five days after the queen has had her litter. This should not be confused with the slight greenish brown discharge which is normal after a cat has given birth. There is increased thirst and vomiting and a high fever. The normal discharge is not accompanied by high temperature and greatly increased thirst.

Treatment: The above symptoms merit a veterinarian's immediate attention.

Pyometra

This condition is usually seen in older (five- to six-year-old) females, especially those queens that have irregular heat periods.

Cause: A pus-producing, abnormal development of the cells lining the womb. The condition occurs in two forms: open and closed.

Open form: A creamy, foul-smelling vaginal discharge; increased thirst; abdominal enlargement (often confused with pregnancy). Since pyometra is not an infectious disease, there is no dramatic rise in body temperature.

Closed form: No visible sign of discharge, since the cervix remains closed and the uterus gradually fills up with pus. This produces a pronounced abdominal enlargement, extreme lethargy, and increased thirst.

Treatment: Both forms of pyometra must be considered serious: they require surgical treatment. Consult a veterinarian.

Vaginal Discharge (See Pyometra)

12

Poisoning

POISONING: GENERAL

Before proceeding to more detailed information re-
garding symptoms and treatments for common poisons, it is
essential to realize that in most instances it is not possible
for the cat owner to diagnose accurately a specific cause of
poisoning from observation of symptoms alone. In the majority of cases, therefore, treatment must be limited to the
general procedure covering all forms of poisoning.

Symptoms: Vomiting; diarrhea; internal hemorrhage;
incoordination; twitching; convulsions; unconsciousness;
coma. These symptoms are also present in many other
conditions. Without additional evidence, therefore, it is
difficult to pinpoint poison as the cause.

Treatment: If there are reasonable grounds to suspect
that a cat has eaten poison, and if the animal is conscious,
induce vomiting as soon as possible. (See Technique for
inducing vomiting below.)

Vomiting is *not* desirable when acid, lead, or other
corrosive poisons have been ingested. If these poisons are

170

suspected, feed up to ¼ pint of olive oil. Subsequent treatment consists of administering the proper antidote (if you can identify the poison) and treating any symptoms as they arise.

Technique for inducing vomiting: The simplest and fastest way to make the animal vomit is to throw ordinary table salt into the back of the cat's mouth (1 teaspoon of salt is sufficient).

Since the symptoms for different poisons are similar, the only way you can tell one from the other is when you have actually seen, or seen evidence of (e.g., an empty can), a particular poison being ingested. If you are not sure, administer what is hopefully known as the universal antidote. (See Universal antidote below.)

If possible, always bring a sample of the suspected poison and a sample of the cat's vomit to the vet along with the patient. If the poison can be determined quickly, much valuable time can be saved.

Universal antidote: Combine 2 parts charcoal (burned toast), 1 part magnesium oxide (milk of magnesia), and 1 part tannic acid (strong tea). Feed the cat 2 teaspoons of the mixture.

If the cat is unconscious: Do not induce vomiting. Take the animal to a vet. Make sure the tongue is out. Prop open the cat's jaw with a spool of thread.

If the cat was in physical contact with toxic or corrosive substances: Wash the affected area with liberal amounts of clean water. Do not use soap.

If the cat is hyperexcited or having convulsions: Prevent the cat from hurting itself by shutting it into a dark, quiet room or closet with no sharp furniture. When the convulsion has passed, administer a simple sedative (e.g., one-half of a 250-mg. Tylenol ® tablet) to calm the cat. (See How to Administer Tablets and Pills.)

Poison on the skin: If a noncorrosive poison has contacted the skin or fur, bathe the affected portions with soap and water. Even if the poison does not burn the skin, it must be removed immediately; otherwise the cat will lick its fur and ingest the poison.

Acid and Alkali Poisoning

Common acid poisons: Sulfuric acid (found in defoliants and car batteries); nitric acid; hydrochloric acid.

Symptoms: Inflamed patches on skin which, when licked, cause burning of the mouth, profuse drooling, and vomiting.

Treatment for acid poisoning: Administer 4 tablespoons of a solution of 2 tablespoons of sodium bicarbonate to 1 pint of water. Force-feed 4 tablespoons of a solution of 1 egg white to ½ pint of milk. (See Force-Feeding.)

Treatment for acid burns: Bathe the affected area with a solution of 2 tablespoons of bicarbonate of soda to 1 pint of water. Seek professional help.

Common alkali poisons: Caustic soda; caustic potash.

Symptoms: Soapy patches on fur; burning of the mouth; profuse drooling; vomiting.

Treatment for alkali poisoning: Administer 2 tablespoons of a mixture of 1/10 pint of vinegar to 1 pint of water. Wash the cat's mouth out with vinegar. Seek professional help.

Treatment for alkali burns: Apply vinegar to alkali burns by pouring directly over the burn, or by saturating a rag with vinegar and applying it to the affected area. Get professional help.

Warning: If poisoning is suspected, do not attempt to induce vomiting by administering emetics, unless you have seen the cat eat the poison. Cats who get acid or alkali poisons on their fur usually try to lick them off, thereby ingesting them and causing the symptoms listed above.

Arsenic Poisoning

Sources: Rat and mouse poisons; ant poisons; insecticides; sheep and cattle dips; around smelting works and mines. Arsenic is also a common impurity found in many chemicals.

Symptoms: Acute arsenic poisoning may lead to death so quickly that there is no time to observe symptoms. Smaller doses of arsenic produce symptoms that include: intense abdominal pain; vomiting; staggering; diarrhea; collapse; coma; death. The cat's breath has a strong garlicky odor.

Treatment: If the cat is conscious, induce vomiting by feeding 2 teaspoons of table salt. (See Emetics/Induced Vomiting.) Force-feed 4 tablespoons of a solution of 2 tablespoons bicarbonate of soda to 1 pint of water. Give the cat an enema with warm, soapy water. (See Enema.) Administer demulcents (substances that soothe the irritated stomach lining), such as milk, or cornstarch and water, mixed to a thin paste.

Insulin Poisoning (Accidental Overdose)

Cause: Diabetic cats receiving insulin treatment at home may be overdosed inadvertently. This usually occurs within an hour after insulin treatment.

Symptoms: Vary from staggering and incoordination to unconsciousness.

Treatment: If the cat is still conscious, give it 5 lumps of sugar. Break the lumps into tablet-sized bits, to make it easier for you to administer and for the cat to swallow. (See How to Administer Tablets and Pills.) (One lump of sugar equals ½ teaspoon of powdered sugar.)

If the cat has lost consciousness, and a veterinarian is not immediately available, mix sugar and water in the amounts given above. Crush the sugar lumps between spoons to make the sugar dissolve faster, and pour a little at a time into the cat's mouth.

Mercury Poisoning

Sources: Antiseptics and fungicides; broken thermometers and barometers; ointments containing mercury.

Symptoms: Early symptoms are vomiting and diarrhea. If death does not occur immediately from shock, these symptoms are followed by ulceration of the mouth and tongue and acute kidney failure.

Treatment: Since the absorption of mercury into the system is very rapid, swift treatment is essential. If the cat's stomach can be emptied within half an hour of ingestion, there is a good chance of recovery. Induce vomiting (See

Emetics/Induced Vomiting), then force-feed raw egg whites and milk. Induce vomiting again.

Phosphorus Poisoning

Sources: Mouse and rat poisons; insecticides; striking surfaces of matchboxes; red-tipped matches; fireworks.

Symptoms: Classic symptoms are staggering, abdominal pain, and vomiting. If phosphorus poisoning is suspected, pay particular attention to the vomit, which will glow in the dark. The cat's breath and vomit will have a garlicky odor.

Following the onset of these symptoms, there is a period of apparent recovery that may last from three to four hours to several days. After this recovery period, the abdominal pain and vomiting recur together with jaundice (a yellowish tinge appears in the eyes and the mucous membranes) and nervous symptoms which, if ignored, will lead to coma and death.

Treatment: Immediate treatment is essential. Induce vomiting. Force-feed a tablespoon of a solution of 1 teaspoon of copper sulfate (available at drugstores) to 1 pint of water. Induce vomiting again.

Administer 4 tablespoons of a solution of 1 teaspoon potassium permanganate (available at drugstores), to 1 pint of water. Give the cat an enema with warm, soapy water. (See Enema.) Do not feed any fatty foods or milk for the next five days.

Sedative Overdose

Sedatives in the form of sleeping pills are often left around by careless owners and are eaten by unwary pets.

Symptoms: The cat will stagger about and appear very drowsy. It will keep falling asleep. There may or may not be an empty pill container to confirm your suspicions, since the animal may have eaten the container along with the pills. Contact a veterinarian.

Treatment: Induce vomiting. Administer stimulants. Cooled strong tea or black coffee should also be given. Keep the animal awake by slapping its face, until the effects wear off.

Strychnine Poisoning

Sources: Mouse, rat, and mole poisons.

Symptoms: The first symptoms of strychnine poisoning are excessive nervousness, restlessness, noticeable twitching of the muscles, and stiff neck. As the condition progresses, these symptoms become more pronounced and convulsions occur: the limbs are extended and the neck is curved upward and backward. During the early stages, these convulsions are sporadic, but they become progressively more frequent until any external stimulus—the slightest noise, or touch, even an air current—will produce them. During the later stage, the iris is widely dilated, covering nearly the whole surface of the eyeball. Death is caused by inability to breathe due to paralysis of the respiratory muscles.

Treatment: If the cat is having convulsions, have the animal anesthetized by a veterinarian. Do not try to take the cat to the vet; you will not make it in time. Have the vet come to the cat.

It is extremely difficult and dangerous to move a convulsing cat. If you attempt to confine it to a closed basket, the cat runs the risk of choking on its vomit. If you must transport the cat, glance inside the box or basket from time to time to make sure this has not happened.

If a vet can be reached by telephone, and if convulsions have not yet begun, get someone to contact the vet while you induce vomiting. After the cat has vomited, force-feed strong cold tea (tannic acid). While waiting for the vet, keep the cat very quiet and insulated from any external stimuli that might trigger convulsions. Place the cat in a quiet, darkened room.

Index

Accidents *(continued)*
  miscarriage, 160
  moving an injured cat, 19–20, 56–57, 106
  overdose of insulin, 138–139, 174
  porcupines, 97
  self-mutilation, 115
  skunks, 97
  slipped disk, 134
  swallowing sharp objects, 79
  traumatic amputation, 125–126
  traumatic hernia (rupture), 114
  See also Poisoning
Acid burns, 94, 172
  inflamed patches on skin, 172
Acid poisoning, 170, 172
  burning of mouth, 172
  drooling, 172
  vomiting, 172
Acid odor of vomit, 156
Acquired deafness, 62
Acute abdomen, 155
Acute middle ear infection. *See* Middle ear
  infection, acute
Acute otitis. *See* Otitis, acute
Afterbirth, 164. *See also* Placenta
Agalactia (inability to give milk), 161
  first litter, 161
  kittens restless and fretful, 161
Airsickness. *See* Motion sickness
Alkali burns, 94, 172–173
  soapy patches on fur, 172
Alkali poisoning, 172
  burning of mouth, 172
  drooling, 172
  vomiting, 172
Allergies, general symptoms of, 135–136
  diarrhea, 135
  running eyes, 135
  skin, red and itching, 135
  swollen lips and eyelids, 135
  vomiting, 135
Allergies of the respiratory tract, 104–105.
  See also Asthma; Hay fever
Allergies of the skin, 82, 86–89
Alopecia. *See* Baldness
Amputation
  frostbite and, 96
  surgical, 125
  traumatic, 125–126
Analgesics, 14
Anal impaction, 31–32, 118
Anemia, 136, 153
  chronic, 136
  lethargy, 136
  pallor of face, 136

  rapid pulse, 136
  shock, 153
Animal bites, 91, 100, 147
Anorectal region
  abnormal stools, 117
  abscess, 114
  bleeding from anus, 118
  blood in stools, 117, 118
  constipation, 118
  diarrhea, 119
  enemas, 31–32
  hard stools, 117
  loose stools, 117, 119
  prolapse of the rectum, 120
  rectal tumors, 118
  soreness, 119
  tapeworms, 121
  worms, 120–121
Anorexia. *See* Appetite, loss of
Anthropomorphism, 14–15
Antibiotics, 15
Antidotes
  for acid and alkali poisoning, 172
  for arsenic poisoning, 173
  for mercury poisoning, 174–175
  for phosphorus poisoning, 175
  for strychnine poisoning, 177
  universal, 171
Antiseptics, mercury poisoning from,
  174–175
Ant poisons, arsenic poisoning from, 173
Anus
  bleeding from, 21, 118
  segments of worms around, 121
  sore, 36, 119
Apathy, 35, 79, 153, 157
Appetite
  excessive, 157
  increased, 138
  loss of, 52, 73, 74, 79, 88, 107, 108, 113,
  139, 157
  reduced, 121
  stimulating a poor, 35, 45, 46, 47, 158
Arsenic poisoning
  abdominal pain, 173
  collapse, 173
  coma, 173
  diarrhea, 173
  garlic odor of breath, 173
  staggering, 173
  treatment for, 173
  vomiting, 156, 173
Arterial wounds
  blood comes out in pumping fashion, 20,
  54